HIGH CHOLESTEROL

This edition first published in Canada in 2007 by Whitecap Books,
351 Lynn Ave., North Vancouver, British Columbia, Canada, V7J 2C4.

www.whitecap.ca

ISBN 1 55285 877 4
ISBN 978 1 55285 877 6

Chief Executive: Juliet Rogers
Publishing Director: Kay Scarlett

Design manager: Vivien Valk
Project manager and editor: Emma Hutchinson
Recipe consultant and nutrition analyst: Susanna Holt
Design concept: Susanne Geppert
Designer: Anthony Vandenberg
Photographers: Jared Fowler and Ian Hofstetter
Stylists: Jane Collins, Katy Holder and Cherise Koch
Food preparation: Joanne Kelly and Alan Wilson
Recipes by: Michelle Earl and members of the Murdoch Books Test Kitchen
Production: Monique Layt

First published in 2007 by Murdoch Books Pty Limited.

Printed by Sing Cheong Printing Co. Ltd. in 2007. PRINTED IN HONG KONG.

The Publisher and stylist would like to thank Dinosaur Designs, Mud Australia, Bison Homewares and IKEA for assistance in the photography of this book.

IMPORTANT: Those who might be at risk from the effects of salmonella poisoning (the elderly, pregnant women, young children and those suffering from immune deficiency diseases) should consult their doctor with any concerns about eating raw eggs.

CONVERSION GUIDE: You may find cooking times vary depending on the oven you are using. For fan-forced ovens, as a general rule, set the oven temperature to 20°C (35°F) lower than indicated in the recipe. We have used 20 ml (4 teaspoon) tablespoon measures. If you are using a 15 ml (3 teaspoon) tablespoon, for most recipes the difference will not be noticeable. However, for recipes using baking powder, gelatine, bicarbonate of soda (baking soda), small amounts of flour and cornflour (cornstarch), add an extra teaspoon for each tablespoon specified.

EATWELLLIVEWELL

with HIGH CHOLESTEROL

Low-cholesterol recipes and tips

Introductory text by Karen Kingham (nutritionist)

whitecap

CONTENTS

LOWER CHOLESTEROL THE HEALTHY WAY

High blood cholesterol is one of the major risk factors for heart disease, which can lead to heart attack or stroke. Simply put, the higher the cholesterol level, the greater the risk. Best estimates rank cardiovascular disease (CVD) as the leading cause of death in the Western world. The expectation is that CVD will become an even greater health problem, along with obesity and diabetes, by the end of the next decade.

The good news in all of this is the lower you get your blood cholesterol, the lower your risk of CVD and the less chance you have of becoming a health statistic.

There is plenty you can do to achieve a lower blood cholesterol level, the most important being improving your diet and lifestyle. Diets to lower cholesterol have come a long way in the last 20 years. Bland high-fibre meals devoid of fat are out, flavoursome and colourful meals using the right fats are in. So take the opportunity to change your life—enjoy the recipes in this book with family and friends, lower your cholesterol and live a longer healthier life.

What is cholesterol?

Cholesterol is a waxy, fatty substance made naturally, in amounts determined by your genetic make-up, by the liver. We all need a certain amount of cholesterol to make hormones, coat our nerve cells so signals travel properly, and form the outer membranes of our body's cells. Cholesterol is not bad for us when we have it in the right amounts.

Our body also gets small amounts of cholesterol from the foods we eat, such as shellfish, meat, chicken, eggs, butter, cheese and whole milk. Foods with saturated and trans fats can upset the body's cholesterol balance by causing your liver to make more cholesterol than it otherwise would.

Because cholesterol is a fat and can't dissolve in the blood it must get to and from the cells via transporters or carriers known as lipoproteins, of which there are two types.

Low-density lipoprotein or LDL cholesterol: This is found in the greatest amounts and is the one you most need to worry about.

LDL's main job is to take cholesterol from the liver to the body cells where it is needed. Too much LDL causes a build-up of cholesterol on the inside of blood vessel walls which is not good for your health.

High-density lipoprotein or HDL cholesterol: This is the cholesterol you want to have more of. HDL tidies up excess cholesterol, picking it up from your blood vessels and taking it back to your liver.

The trouble with too much LDL cholesterol

Too much LDL cholesterol in your blood causes the excess to be deposited in the blood vessels. Over time, the cholesterol along with other substances builds up in the vessel walls causing them to narrow and then harden—think of the sludge you might get clogging up your drain pipes at home. This process is known as atherosclerosis.

Cholesterol deposited in the blood vessels is also more susceptible to a process known as oxidation. When LDL is oxidized it becomes more irritating to the blood vessel causing inflammation, which then accelerates the process of atherosclerosis.

Depending on your genes, diet and lifestyle, atherosclerosis can start as early as childhood and can become quite advanced by the time you reach middle age.

Atherosclerosis is involved in the progression of a number of diseases:

- **Coronary heart disease** occurs when the blood vessels to the heart are affected by atherosclerosis and can lead to angina (chest pain) or a heart attack.
- **Cerebrovascular disease** is caused by narrowing or blockages in blood vessels to the brain and can result in a stroke.
- **Peripheral vascular disease** is the result of narrowing or blockage of the blood

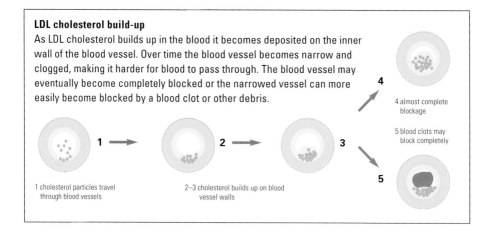

LDL cholesterol build-up

As LDL cholesterol builds up in the blood it becomes deposited on the inner wall of the blood vessel. Over time the blood vessel becomes narrow and clogged, making it harder for blood to pass through. The blood vessel may eventually become completely blocked or the narrowed vessel can more easily become blocked by a blood clot or other debris.

4 almost complete blockage

5 blood clots may block completely

1 cholesterol particles travel through blood vessels

2–3 cholesterol builds up on blood vessel walls

vessels in parts of the body other than the brain or heart, such as the legs, arms, stomach, kidneys or other organs.

These diseases of the heart and blood vessels caused by atherosclerosis are collectively known as CVD, the number one cause of death for men and women in Western countries.

Your cholesterol target

If your blood cholesterol is high your doctor will give you advice on the best level to aim for. Regardless of how high your blood cholesterol is, the lower you get LDL cholesterol the better off you'll be.

The National Heart Foundation of Australia and the Cardiac Society of Australia and New Zealand recommends you keep blood cholesterol levels in the following range*:

Total cholesterol	less than 4.0 mmol/L
LDL cholesterol	less than 2.0 mmol/L
HDL cholesterol	more than 1.0 mmol/L

*Depending upon where in the world you live these may differ.

What affects cholesterol levels?

Living in the Western world there are a number of factors that may cause your cholesterol to rise. Some of these you can change, some you can't.

These are the factors you can't change

- **Your age and gender:** blood cholesterol tends to rise as we get older and is usually higher in men than women until after the menopause. A woman's cholesterol may quickly catch up to that of men of a similar age once the menopause is over.
- **Your inheritance:** high blood cholesterol can run in families and your genes may also put you at greater risk.

How common is high cholesterol?

Thirty to fifty per cent of adults in Western countries have high blood cholesterol. Despite knowing about the harmful effects of high cholesterol and understanding how easy it can be to lower it, the numbers of people with high blood cholesterol has changed little in some countries since the 1980s.

These are the factors you can change

- **Your weight:** the world's population has become dramatically heavier over the past 20 years. Rates of overweight and obesity in Western nations have climbed to as much as 60 per cent. And as our weight increases so too is the likelihood that LDL cholesterol will be higher and HDL will be lower than is ideal.
- **Your diet:** eating a diet high in saturated fat is one of the most significant causes of high LDL cholesterol. Major sources of saturated fat in our diet include butter, cream, cheese and other full-fat dairy products, the fat associated with meat and poultry (especially from skin), sausages, salami and other processed meats. Significant amounts are also found in many baked goods (biscuits (cookies), cakes, pies, pastries), fried take-away foods and snack foods (chocolate, potato crisps, corn chips and cheese-flavoured snacks).
- **How much you move:** being more physically active will not only lower your LDL cholesterol but improve your risk-factor profile for CVD by lowering blood pressure, reducing insulin resistance, helping with weight control and improving mental health. Being more physically active will also lower your risk of developing type 2 diabetes, osteoporosis, obesity, breast and colon cancer, and depression.

What about triglycerides?

If you've had a cholesterol test, it is likely that the results included information about triglycerides: these are a type of fat found in your blood. Triglycerides come from the fats in the food you eat and are also made in the body—especially if you eat too many kilojoules—your body then turns them into triglycerides (fat).

The link between high triglycerides and CVD remains uncertain, but when triglycerides are high, your risk of heart problems usually rises, especially if your LDL cholesterol is also high.

Triglyceride levels tend to be high if you smoke, drink alcohol to excess, are obese, don't exercise enough or eat too many refined carbohydrates. Type 2 diabetes and liver and kidney diseases also increase your chances of having high triglycerides, as can your genes.

Ideally, you should aim to keep your triglycerides less than 1.5 mmol/L. Do this by following the advice given in this book, giving up smoking, drinking less alcohol and eating less refined and more wholegrain and low-GI carbohydrates.

Risk factors for cardiovascular disease

If you have high blood cholesterol, have you considered how high your risk of CVD is and what your chances are of having a heart attack or stroke? These are important questions that everyone with high cholesterol should know the answers to. The most accurate answer—your risk in percentage terms—is best calculated by your doctor. However, you can get a rough idea by considering how many of these risk factors apply to you:

- High total and LDL cholesterol
- Low HDL cholesterol
- High triglycerides
- Cigarette smoking
- High blood pressure (for example, over 140/90 mmHg)
- Overweight and obesity
- Inactivity
- Diabetes or pre-diabetes
- Stress, depression and social isolation
- Aged over 45 years
- Family history of heart disease (parent or sibling affected at less than 60 years of age)
- Kidney transplant or kidney disease
- Aboriginal or Torres Strait Islander descent
- Maori or Pacific Islander descent
- Asian or from the Indian subcontinent
- African or Mexican American

   In general, the higher your LDL cholesterol level and the more risk factors you have, the greater your chances of developing CVD and having a heart attack or stroke. Fortunately by living a healthier life you can make a real difference to many of your risk factors. In short, give up smoking, take charge of your diet and get out of the house and move more.

The issue of weight

Being overweight increases your risk of high cholesterol and CVD as well as many other health problems. Overweight is defined as having a body mass index (BMI) of 25 or more. If you know your weight and height you can work out your BMI:

$$BMI = \frac{Weight\ (kg)}{Height\ (m)^2}$$

Maintaining a healthy weight
Following is a list of all the good reasons why you should aim to keep your weight down using a heart healthy diet and regular exercise:

Heart health benefits
- Lower LDL cholesterol
- Higher HDL cholesterol
- Lower triglycerides
- Lower blood pressure
- Improve insulin resistance and control blood glucose if you have diabetes
- Reduce your risk of CVD

General health benefits
- Reduce risk of type 2 diabetes
- Lower risk of some cancers
- Improve sleep apnoea
- Reduce joint pain in arthritis
- Control gout
- Lower risk of gall bladder disease
- Improve asthma
- Relieve reflux
- Improve fertility

For most people their BMI is a good indicator of body fat levels and health risks. But there are some—such as athletes and those of some ethnic groups (for example, Pacific Islanders and South-East Asians)—who are the exception.

Where on your body you store your fat makes a big difference to your CVD risk. Fat stored around your tummy (apple shapes) puts you at greater risk than fat stored on your hips and thighs (pear shapes).

Checking your waist size is easy using a tape measure at the level of your belly button. Women should aim for a waist less than 80 cm (31½ in) and men less than 94 cm (37 in). A waist size greater than this makes you a bigger candidate for a heart attack or stroke.

Healthier eating habits to lower blood cholesterol

Better eating habits and a healthier lifestyle—which includes being more active as well as giving up smoking—are two of the biggest steps you can take to lower your blood cholesterol. This is why your doctor will usually give you a chance with these before prescribing you any medication. These changes are also the best way to avoid getting high cholesterol.

Once you have commenced your plan to lower cholesterol don't forget to visit your doctor and keep track of your progress. Anyone with high cholesterol and at high risk of CVD should have their blood cholesterol checked every year. The benefits of the changes you will make are well proven, but there's no better motivator than to see improvements in your LDL and HDL cholesterol for yourself.

Fast food, be it take-away or made at home from highly processed ingredients, is high in saturated fat, low in fibre and contains fewer vitamins and minerals. When eaten regularly, this sort of food slows you down and makes you more likely to suffer health problems, particularly high cholesterol.

Women take special care

Cardiovascular disease claims five times the lives that breast cancer does. Yet, high blood cholesterol and CVD are often dismissed by women as being male problems. Protective female hormones give women an extra 10 to 15 years of good cardiovascular health compared to men. However, blood cholesterol levels can rise significantly after the menopause. With these extra years 'up your sleeve' a valuable opportunity exists to take care of yourself and intercept the consequences of menopause to live a longer, healthier life.

Advancing knowledge in nutrition tells us that while we go forwards in some things, in others we go back. For the health of your heart and blood vessels going back to basics and embracing natural unprocessed foods is what you need. This doesn't mean a return to the bland, high-fibre, low-fat diets of the 1980s. Instead it means going back to more traditional foods such as:

- wholegrains, legumes and fresh fruit and vegetables for their antioxidants, phytochemicals and low-GI carbohydrates
- nuts, seeds and more fish for their healthier fats
- lean meat, chicken, seafood and low fat dairy for vital protein.

An abundance of foods have proven heart health benefits and many will be discussed in the following pages. But no single food will keep cholesterol at bay. Success is only possible by including as many heart-friendly foods in your diet as possible. Heart healthy eating habits are additive. If you can follow all of the advice given here there is the potential to drop blood cholesterol by as much as a 30 per cent—better than some medications prescribed by your doctor.

Don't despair if you don't manage to follow all the advice given here. Start with the most important—cutting down on your saturated fat. Use our guides and tips to track saturated fat down and remove it from your diet. Once you have made this change successfully choose another, then another, until you have made them all. If you are finding it hard to achieve our advice or if you have diabetes, kidney disease or any other serious medical problems, seek the advice of a dietitian. This will ensure your eating plan is in tune with your lifestyle and meets your individual health needs making a lower cholesterol easier to achieve.

Cut the bad fat

Just as there is good and bad blood cholesterol, there are good and bad fats. Rather than ridding your diet of all fat, the best thing you can do to get your cholesterol down is to achieve the right balance of good and bad fats.

Saturated fat is the biggest culprit for raising your LDL cholesterol level. These fats are usually of animal origin (except for palm oil and coconut fat). Trans fats come a close second in cholesterol-raising ability. Trans fats occur naturally in some foods of animal origin such as beef, lamb and dairy foods. They are also made when liquid vegetable oils are turned into hard fats (margarines and solid frying fats) for commercial food production. This process is known as hydrogenation or partial hydrogenation.

Major sources of trans fats include crackers, biscuits (cookies), doughnuts, corn and potato crisps, margarine, hot chips and other commercially produced fried foods—anything prepared using hydrogenated or partially hydro-genated oils. Some countries have higher levels of trans fats in their foods than others, but this is changing as governments become more aware of the health threat they pose and place pressure on food industries to lower the amount of trans fats in the foods they produce. Cutting back on saturated and trans fats and using healthier monounsaturated and polyunsaturated fats will lower LDL and raise HDL cholesterol. Our easy-to-read table on the right lets you find these bad fats so you can make better choices when you shop.

Make sure you include a good balance of polyunsaturated and monounsaturated fats in your diet by thinking about variety:

- Use a range of oils in your meal preparations—sunflower or canola for baking, extra virgin olive, macadamia or walnut for salad dressings, peanut or sesame for Asian stir fries.
- Spread your bread with margarine spreads made from vegetable oils, avocado, low fat dips and mayonnaise, peanut butter, ricotta or cottage cheese.

Where is the bad fat?
Ridding your diet of saturated and trans fats takes time and practice. Consider the following tips for ousting these bad fellows from your life:

- Avoid butter, lard, cream, sour cream, coconut milk or cream and hard cooking margarines
- Choose lean cuts of meat and trim any remaining fat before cooking
- Choose skinless cuts of chicken or remove the skin before eating
- Eat cheese less often and choose lower fat varieties
- Avoid high fat processed deli meats like devon, chicken loaf and salami
- Use low or reduced fat milks, yoghurts, ice creams and custard
- Avoid deep fried takeaway foods, pies, sausage rolls and pasties
- Choose tomato based pasta sauces over creamy types
- Save commercial biscuits (cookies), cakes, muffins, pastries and puddings for special occasions
- Cut back on high fat snack foods, such as chocolate bars, crisps and savoury crackers
- Cook with low fat methods: steaming, grilling, dry frying, baking and barbecuing

Moderate dietary cholesterol

So, what about dietary cholesterol? The consensus is while it's still important to keep cholesterol down, it's not as big a taboo as it once was.

The body of research now shows cholesterol from food can have little impact on your blood cholesterol levels, especially when your overall diet is good. Eggs, prawns and other crustaceans are also low in saturated fat and can be good sources of heart friendly omega-3 fats.

Moderation in dietary cholesterol does, however, remain the key. Expert opinion varies, but limiting your intake of eggs to three to four a week and having the occasional meal of prawns cooked without added fat is unlikely to do most people with high cholesterol any harm. If you have familial hypercholesterolaemia or a very high risk of heart disease you are likely to be an exception to this advice and should take steps to be more strict with your cholesterol intake.

Health authorities recommend keeping total dietary cholesterol intake under 200–300 mg a day. Check our cholesterol ready reckoner on page 19 to see what that means for you.

Balance your kilojoules

We live in a world where upsizing and 'meal deals' are commonplace, quick-fix fad diets are bestsellers, and gadgets to save time and energy abound. It's no wonder we are in the midst of an obesity epidemic. Strategies to stop weight gain are essential in any heart-friendly eating plan and the most important of these are portion and kilojoule control. The sums to support this are simple, eat too much food and kilojoules and you put on weight, eat less food and kilojoules and you lose weight—or at the very least you won't gain. Despite the promises of diet books, there are no special foods or ways of eating that will change this basic equation. Physical activity is the only factor you can add to tip the balance in your favour.

Cutting back on your kilojoules means focusing on foods that give you more for less—foods with more nutrients but less kilojoules. Give foods like crisps, commercial cakes, pastries and biscuits, sweets, soft drinks and high-fat savoury crackers the flick and eat more fruit, vegetables, wholegrain breads and cereals, lean meat, fish, nuts and seeds.

Watching the total amount of fat you eat also makes it easier to balance your kilojoules. A no-fat diet is no good for lowering cholesterol (it's the balance of good fats and bad fats that counts) or losing weight for that matter (it just makes your diet unpalatable and hard to maintain), but eating less saturated fat will rid your diet of many unhealthy and surplus kilojoules. Re-visit our tips for cutting back on saturated fat on page 15 to make sure you target the right ones.

Controlling portion sizes will also mean fewer kilojoules. Try eating only the recommended serve of your cereal at breakfast—1⅓ cups of ready-to-eat cereal, ½ cup of natural muesli or 1 cup of cooked porridge—use a smaller sized plate or bowl for meals or order an entrée-sized meal if you must have a dessert when eating out. If you want seconds go for another serve of salad or vegetables rather than the meat or the pasta/rice. Another trick to keeping portions in check is to divide up your plate at meal time—allow a quarter of the plate for your protein (such as meat), a quarter for your carbohydrate and the remaining half for salad or vegetables.

Choosing your carbohydrates wisely will also help with portion control. Select higher fibre, low-GI carbohydrates like grainy bread, pasta, oat-based breakfast cereals, sweet potato, corn, legumes and temperate fruits. Their slower digestion and absorption will keep you feeling fuller and satisfied for longer and make you less likely to snack before your next meal. Their soluble fibre also helps lower your blood cholesterol.

Statistics tell us that if you are overweight you may never achieve your healthy weight goals despite your best attempts. If you do succeed, it can slip away again within three to five years with creeping weight gains. However, don't let this deter you.

Any weight you lose will make you healthier and fitter. You only need a weight loss of around five to ten per cent to make a positive difference to your cholesterol.

If you need more help with your weight and diet plan, visit a dietitian. They can help you with a heart-friendly eating plan to help you keep the kilos off.

Seek out antioxidants

Free radicals cause damage to your body—known as oxidation—which leads to ageing and disease. When LDL cholesterol is oxidized by free radicals it becomes stickier and is more likely to take part in the process of atherosclerosis—this makes it more dangerous. You can prevent oxidation of LDL cholesterol by making sure you eat plenty of foods rich in antioxidants. Antioxidants are natural chemicals found in food that protect your body from damage by free radicals. Some antioxidants are also nutrients—think of vitamin C, E and selenium, while others are simply naturally occurring plant chemicals known as phytochemicals, such as the flavonoids, catechins and anthocyanins.

Colour is a good sign of a food's health potential and most of the foods richest in antioxidant ability are also rich in colour. Think of berries, citrus, cherries, plums, spinach and other green leafy vegetables, broccoli, red capsicum and beetroot.

Other antioxidant-rich foods include tea, red wine, chocolate, extra virgin olive oil, nuts and herbs.

Taking antioxidants out of food and putting them into a supplement can in some cases do you no good and may even do you harm. The safest and most effective way to get antioxidants is through food. What would you enjoy more, a bowl of fresh raspberries and a few squares of premium dark chocolate or a supplement pill?

Enjoy more plant foods

Research the world over reveals that people who eat the most fruit and vegetables are the healthiest and longest living of all. With most rich in cholesterol-lowering soluble fibre and sterols, fruits and vegetables are also packed with heart-protective vitamins, minerals and antioxidants. With maximum nutrition, plant foods come at a very low kilojoule cost so are a great choice when you need to control your weight. To get the most from fruit and vegetables eat by the rainbow. Choose at least two serves of fruit and five serves of vegetables each day, selecting the brightest and most colourful types to get maximum benefits.

Where's the cholesterol?	
Food	Cholesterol mg
Kidney, 100 g	500
Liver, 100 g	400
Egg, 1 large	210
Lobster, 100 g	150
Prawns, 100 g	110

Legumes are another important plant food. Be they fresh, dried or canned, legumes (for example, beans, split peas, chickpeas and lentils) are excellent sources of soluble fibre and low in saturated fat. Legumes are low in GI and rich in heart-friendly antioxidants that protect cholesterol from the oxidative damage that makes it more likely to clog up your arteries.

To reap the health rewards of legumes, incorporate them into at least a couple of meals a week. They make a great vegetarian alternative in curries (chickpeas) and Mexican dishes (kidney beans) but also serve up well at breakfast. You can also try cutting back the meat a little and adding them to stews and soups or using them to lower the GI of grains like rice and couscous.

Finally, don't forget nuts and seeds. Formerly considered to be off limits for anyone wanting a healthier diet, nuts and seeds have been given the thumbs up. While high in fats (the healthy kind) and kilojoules, they are also rich in fibre, healthy fats and heart-protective nutrients like vitamin E, folate, magnesium and copper.

A small handful of unsalted nuts (raw, toasted or dry roasted) as a daily snack, or nuts and seeds added to salads, pasta or breakfast cereals are a good habit for a healthier heart. If you need to lose weight, include them only occasionally—up to a couple of times a week and always stop at just a small handful. Reassuringly, studies show those who eat nuts regularly are more likely to be a healthy weight.

Eat more fibre

Fibre is your friend when you need to get cholesterol down. Unfortunately most of us aren't friendly enough with fibre. Our intakes are often way down compared with the 25–30 g of fibre a day that's recommended.

Two types of fibre exist in food—soluble and insoluble. Both offer you plenty of health benefits, but it's the soluble fibre that directly affects blood cholesterol. Found in oats, barley, psyllium, legumes and some fruit and vegetables, soluble fibre forms a gel-like substance in your intestine that binds up cholesterol and stops your body absorbing it. Increase the soluble fibre in your diet by adding psyllium husk or oat, barley or rice bran to your breakfast cereal or baking recipes as well as making sure you eat enough fruit, vegetables and legumes.

Foods made from the whole of the grain—known as wholegrain foods—are also rich in fibre (both soluble and insoluble), low in GI and packed with essential nutrients and antioxidants. The combination of goodies found in wholegrains is responsible for their undisputed ability to protect not only from CVD but also diabetes, overweight and certain types of cancer.

Get the most out of these heart-friendly foods by making half of all the grain foods you eat wholegrain. If you are aiming for six serves of cereal foods a day then at least three serves should be wholegrain. The problem is, most of us are lucky to even make one serve, let alone three.

What fat is that?

Fat	Where will you find it?
Saturated fats	butter, cream, palm oil, coconut milk and cream, fried foods and take-aways, fat on meat and skin on chicken, full-fat dairy foods, deli meats and most commercial cakes, pastries, confectionery and biscuits
Monounsaturated fats	olives and olive oil, avocados, peanuts and peanut oil, canola oil, macadamia nuts, hazelnuts, pecan nuts, cashews and almonds
Omega-6 polyunsaturated fats	sunflower, safflower, soya bean, sesame, cottonseed and grape seed oils, pine nuts and Brazil nuts
Omega-3 polyunsaturated fats	oily types of fish; herring, sardine, mackerel, salmon and tuna; walnuts, canola oil, linseeds (flax seeds) and linseed oil, lean red meat and a range of fortified commercial foods
Trans fats	margarines and fat spreads (some countries have less trans fats in these than others—check labels), deep-fried fast food, commercial cakes, pastries, pies and biscuits—look for the words hydrogenated or partially hydrogenated fats on food labels

Wholegrain foods aren't just 'whole' grains like brown rice and whole-wheat. Wholegrain foods can be processed and still retain the important components of the wholegrain. Boost your daily serves of wholegrain foods by:

- using wholemeal (whole-wheat) flour instead of white
- snacking on whole-wheat crackers or popcorn
- enjoying oats, natural muesli or whole-wheat cereals at breakfast
- choosing wholegrain or wholemeal breads
- trying brown rice or barley as a change from white rice
- choosing wholemeal rather than white pasta

Eat more fish

Fish, especially oily fish contain healthy unsaturated fats known as long chain omega-3s. Omega-3 fats are a type of polyunsaturated fat that are essential to our health and must come from our diet. These fats protect the heart and blood vessels by lowering triglycerides, keeping the heart beating regularly (preventing arrhythmias), maintaining more elastic blood vessels, lessening the risk of blood clots by keeping the blood more free flowing, and calming inflammation.

To benefit most from omega-3, include oily fish at least twice a week. Highest concentrations of omega-3 can be found in sardines, salmon, mackerel, tuna, trevally, trout, pilchards and flathead. All fish, even the oily varieties, are low in saturated fat and so are a healthy choice at any meal.

It makes no difference if your fish is fresh or canned. The convenience of canned fish makes it perfect for busy lives and those who don't live near the sea. Take care to avoid fish packed in brine—you don't need the extra salt. Instead, look for canned fish packed in spring water and check the label for those with the most omega-3.

Consider plant sterols

Plant sterols are found naturally in plant-based foods such as vegetable oils, legumes, fruit, nuts and seeds. Able to reduce the amount of cholesterol your body absorbs

21

from your intestine, plant sterols ultimately lower blood cholesterol. A typical Western diet won't have enough plant sterols to make a difference to blood cholesterol but one that includes foods enriched with plant sterols will.

Depending upon where in the world you live you may find margarine spreads, milk, yoghurt and even breakfast cereals enriched with plant sterols. For blood cholesterol benefits you need to eat 2–3 g of plant sterols every day.

As a rule, three serves of a sterol-enriched food will give you enough plant sterols for the cholesterol-lowering benefits—check product packaging to be sure.

> **Up your oats**
> Oats are a food with a proven record for lowering cholesterol because of a soluble fibre known as beta glucan. But just don't eat any oats (though they are all good for you), go for the slower cooking, old fashioned varieties such as traditional, steel-cut or scotch oats, which will have a lower GI and more beta glucan than quick-cook and instant varieties.

Sterol-enriched foods can't be expected to take the place of a healthy diet that is low in saturated fat. However, the weight of evidence is behind them and Heart Associations around the world recommend plant sterol-enriched foods be considered as part of a cholesterol lowering diet.

Keep salt down

Although rising blood pressure as we age appears to be inevitable in the Western world, there are steps you can take to keep blood pressure in check. Losing weight, drinking less alcohol, being active and eating more fruit and vegetables will all help, as will cutting down on salt.

Around 75 per cent of the salt we eat comes from processed foods. So simply avoiding salt in cooking or on the table is not enough. To get your salt intake down to healthier levels take care with what you bring home from the supermarket. Look for reduced-salt or no-added-salt varieties of the regular foods you buy, such as margarine spreads, tinned tomatoes, tomato paste, tomato sauce, cracker biscuits, peanut butter, cheese, bread, cooking stocks and sauces.

Avoiding obviously salty foods such as bacon, ham, olives, hard cheeses, canned fish in brine, salted nuts and crisps will also help, as will using liberal amounts of fresh and dried herbs and spices to boost flavour and make the transition easier. Herbs and spices have added benefits besides the extra flavour—they are rich sources of health protective phytochemicals and antioxidants.

Drink alcohol in moderation

Research suggests that moderate alcohol consumption—a little regularly—can protect your heart and blood vessels. This is apparently the reason the French have such a good record for heart health. In Australia, moderate or low-risk alcohol consumption is defined as no more than four standard drinks a day for men and two for women with one or two alcohol free days each week. However, research shows the optimum amount for heart health may be even less. The American Heart Association recommends no more than two drinks a day for men and one for women in its latest dietary and lifestyle recommendations to reduce CVD.

It also appears not to matter what you drink provided it is alcoholic. Beer, spirits, white wine or red, they all do a similar job—raising good HDL and keeping your blood flowing freely. Red wine with its antioxidants may offer a little extra benefit, but when all is said and done choose what you enjoy most and keep your intake modest.

Unfortunately, alcohol is a double-edged sword. Loaded with kilojoules, alcohol is not good for your weight and too much raises your blood pressure and triglycerides—all of which increase your risk of heart disease. In excess, alcohol is also responsible for liver disease, some forms of cancer and early death by misadventure. For these reasons, if you don't already drink, don't start just to lower your risk of cardiovascular disease.

If you find it hard to just have one or two drinks try to:

- reduce your thirst with water or diet drinks before you drink alcohol
- choose low alcohol beer
- alternate alcoholic and non-alcoholic drinks
- dilute alcoholic drinks such as wine with soda, or a beer with diet lemonade.

Final words on lifestyle to lower cholesterol

Despite the fact that this is a cookbook, advice about lowering cholesterol and improving heart health is not complete without mentioning the importance of a healthy lifestyle. Giving up smoking and becoming more physically active are essential for keeping your heart—and the rest of your body—healthy.

Sitting around like a couch potato makes you twice as likely to die of a heart attack as someone who regularly exercises. Continuing to smoke means a heart attack is up to six times more likely for you than for someone who doesn't smoke.

Taking up the lifestyle challenge offers impressive results: within just one year of quitting smoking, heart disease risk drops by 50 per cent, and if you are overweight but fit, your risk of early death drops to around one-third that of your equally heavy but unfit peers. What's more, those that have the most to gain from moving more are those who are currently doing the least.

Contact your local quit-smoking services to start the ball rolling toward going smoke free. These services can give you the best advice about when and how to start to quit plus support and motivation to keep you going once you are on your way.

Before tackling your fitness regimen discuss your plans with your doctor. This is especially important if you haven't exercised regularly for a while or have other health problems. When you have the all-clear aim to build up to 30 minutes of moderate intensity activity on most, if not all days of the week. Moderate intensity means you are breathing a little harder, but you can still chat with a friend.

If you are new to the whole exercise thing, consider a few sessions with a personal trainer or exercise physiologist. They can design you a program that suits your health needs best.

Your 30 minutes doesn't have to be continuous either. Research shows three lots of 10 minute sessions offer the same benefits as one 30-minute session. Thirty minutes is also the bare minimum you need for health. If you are up to it, and can do more, then there are only greater health benefits to gain. To lose weight you need to do at least 60 minutes of exercise a day.

Consider these ways to be more physically active in your life:

- invest in a pedometer and work towards more steps (or 7500–10 000 steps a day if you are up to the challenge)
- take the stairs rather than the lift or escalator
- park a little further away from the entrance to your work or the shopping mall
- walk to get the paper rather than taking the car
- get up to turn the TV off rather than using the remote
- make a regular date with a friend to go for a walk
- hop on your bike and go for a ride or invest in an exercise bike—you can get at least 30–60 minutes just watching your favourite TV show
- join a water aerobics group—this is good if you have joint problems or are very overweight
- take up a physical hobby like line dancing, yoga, swimming, tennis or golf
- enjoy active weekends with family and friends: go to the park for a picnic and a game of cricket or Frisbee, go bushwalking or take a visit to the city for some sight-seeing.

How to use this book

The tested recipes in this book have been selected to offer you a range of heart-healthy meals and snacks that can be enjoyed by everyone. Switching the whole family to healthier eating means everyone benefits—especially children. Good habits are learnt young—just don't forget children under 2 years should continue with their full-fat dairy foods. From 2 years, introduce the lower fat products the rest of the family use.

There are recipes for everyday meals as well as special occasions and all aim for less saturated fat. To push the benefits of these recipes further we have included low-salt, high-fibre, low-GI and wholegrain ingredients wherever possible. We have also tried to include more heart-protective foods such as oats, legumes, nuts, brightly coloured fruits and vegetables, and fish, so you get the most for your heart and blood vessels from each recipe.

Disclaimer

The information in this book is intended to provide people with high cholesterol, and people who care for them, with general advice about healthy low-cholesterol eating (accurate at the time of printing). This advice may not be sufficient for some people with multiple health problems or serious complications. It is not intended to replace any advice given to you by a qualified doctor or other mainstream health professional. It is important that high cholesterol is diagnosed by a doctor, using standard diagnostic tests (such as blood tests). Neither the author nor the publishers can be held responsible for claims arising from the inappropriate use or incorrect interpretation of any of the dietary advice described in this book.

BREAKFAST

MUESLI BOOST

GET YOURSELF OFF TO AN ENERGY-FUELLED START TO THE DAY WITH THIS NUTRITIOUS MUESLI—RICH IN CARBOHYDRATE, FIBRE, B-GROUP VITAMINS, BETA-CAROTENE, POTASSIUM AND MAGNESIUM.

30 g (1 oz/⅓ cup) flaked almonds
200 g (7 oz/2 cups) rolled (porridge) oats
60 g (2¼ oz/1 cup) processed bran cereal
40 g (1½ oz/⅓ cup) rye flakes
40 g (1½ oz/¼ cup) pepitas
   (pumpkin seeds)
2 tbsp sunflower seeds
1 tbsp linseeds (flax seeds)
90 g (3¼ oz/¾ cup) sultanas
   (golden raisins)

185 g (6½ oz/1 cup) chopped dried apricots
90 g (3¼ oz/½ cup) chopped dried pear
low-fat honey-flavoured yoghurt or skim
   milk, to serve

PREP TIME: 10 MINUTES
COOKING TIME: 5 MINUTES
SERVES 6

Preheat the oven to 160°C (315°F/Gas 2–3). Put the almonds on a baking tray in a single layer and toast in the oven for 5 minutes, or until golden. Remove and set aside.

Put the rolled oats, processed bran cereal, rye flakes, pepitas, sunflower seeds and linseeds in a bowl, then stir well to combine. Add the sultanas, apricots and pears as well as the toasted almonds.

Serve with low-fat honey-flavoured yoghurt or skim milk.

HINT:
• Any remaining muesli can be kept in an airtight container for up to 2 weeks.

nutrition per serve: Energy 1814 kJ (433 Cal); Fat 11.8 g; Saturated fat 1.5 g; Protein 11.2 g; Carbohydrate 65.9 g; Fibre 13.1 g; Cholesterol 0 mg; Sodium 61 mg

BIRCHER MUESLI

This delicious muesli, with the added benefit of fresh fruit, is a great alternative to regular muesli. It's rich in carbohydrate and contains most vitamins and minerals.

300 g (10½ oz/3 cups) rolled (porridge) oats
250 ml (9 fl oz/1 cup) low-fat milk
90 g (3¼ oz/⅓ cup) low-fat plain yoghurt
100 ml (3½ fl oz) orange juice
3 tbsp sugar
125 g (4½ oz/½ cup) low-fat plain yoghurt, extra
2 apples, grated

2 cups mixed seasonal fresh fruit (banana, peach, apricot, melon, apple, strawberries)
honey, to serve (optional)

Prep time: 15 minutes + 4 hours refrigeration
Cooking time: Nil
Serves 6

Put the oats, milk, yoghurt, orange juice and sugar in a bowl and mix together well. Cover and refrigerate for 4 hours, or overnight. Serve with the extra yoghurt, grated apple and fresh fruit of your choice. Drizzle with a little honey, if desired.

HINT:
• You can also add 60 g (2¼ oz/½ cup) slivered almonds, if you like. This will increase the fat and energy content, but the fat will be mostly the unsaturated type.

nutrition per serve: Energy 1277 kJ (305 Cal); Fat 4.5 g; Saturated fat 0.8 g; Protein 10.3 g; Carbohydrate 52.8 g; Fibre 5.5 g; Cholesterol 4 mg; Sodium 55 mg

MIXED BERRY COUSCOUS

185 g (6½ oz/1 cup) instant couscous

500 ml (17 fl oz/2 cups) unsweetened
apple and blackcurrant juice

1 cinnamon stick

250 g (9 oz/2 cups) raspberries

255 g (9 oz/1⅔ cups) blueberries

250 g (9 oz/1⅔ cups) strawberries, hulled
and halved

2 tsp lime or lemon zest, plus extra,
to serve

1 tbsp finely shredded mint

200 g (7 oz) low-fat plain or fruit-flavoured
yoghurt

2 tbsp pure maple syrup

PREP TIME: 10 MINUTES + STANDING +
REFRIGERATION TIME

COOKING TIME: 5 MINUTES

SERVES 4

Put the couscous in a bowl. Pour the apple and blackcurrant juice into a small saucepan and add the cinnamon stick. Bring to the boil, then remove from the heat and pour over the couscous. Cover with plastic wrap and leave to stand for 5 minutes, or until the liquid has been absorbed. Remove the cinnamon stick. Refrigerate.

Separate the couscous grains with a fork, add the berries, lime zest and mint, and gently fold through. Spoon the mixture into 4 bowls. Top with a large dollop of plain or fruit-flavoured yoghurt and drizzle with the maple syrup. Serve chilled.

HINT:
• You can make this dish with many other great fruit combinations, including orange juice and dried fruits or fresh mango, peach, pear and apple.

THIS TASTY LOW-GI BREAKFAST IS
PACKED WITH FRESH SUMMER
FRUIT AND ZESTY SPICES. IT IS A
GOOD SOURCE OF VITAMIN C AND
RICH IN ANTIOXIDANTS.

nutrition per serve: Energy 1525 kJ (364 Cal)
Fat 0.8 g
Saturated fat 0.1 g
Protein 11.2 g
Carbohydrate 73.2 g
Fibre 6.6 g
Cholesterol 2 mg
Sodium 58 mg

PORRIDGE WITH STEWED RHUBARB

INCLUDING RHUBARB IN THIS PORRIDGE MAKES THIS BREAKFAST EVEN MORE NUTRITIOUS THAN REGULAR PORRIDGE—ADDING VITAMIN C, CALCIUM, POTASSIUM AND DIETARY FIBRE.

DRY PORRIDGE MIX
600 g (1 lb 5 oz/6 cups) rolled
  (porridge) oats
55 g (2 oz/½ cup) rolled rice flakes
60 g (2¼ oz/½ cup) rolled barley
60 g (2¼ oz/½ cup) rolled rye
30 g (1 oz/¼ cup) millet flakes

STEWED RHUBARB
350 g (12 oz) rhubarb, trimmed and washed
100 g (3½ oz/½ cup) soft brown sugar
¼ tsp ground mixed spice
low-fat yoghurt, to serve

PREP TIME: 15 MINUTES
COOKING TIME: 30 MINUTES
SERVES 4

Put all the porridge ingredients in a large bowl and mix together well. The dry mix makes about 8 cups or enough for 16 serves. Store in a large airtight container for up to 2 months.

To make enough porridge for 4 serves, put 2 cups porridge mixture in a saucepan with 1.25 litres (44 fl oz/5 cups) water. Bring to the boil, then reduce the heat and simmer, stirring frequently, over a medium heat for 15 minutes, or until the porridge is thick. If it is too thick, add a little skim milk or water.

Meanwhile, to make the stewed rhubarb, chop the rhubarb into 2 cm (¾ in) lengths. Put in a saucepan with the sugar, mixed spice and 250 ml (9 fl oz/1 cup) water. Slowly bring to the boil, stirring to dissolve the sugar, then reduce the heat and simmer for 10 minutes, stirring often. Serve hot or cold with the porridge.

HINTS:
• The cooking time of the porridge will decrease considerably if you use quick-cooking oats (one-minute oats). Check the labels on the packets before purchase. However, quick-cooking oats have a higher GI value than slower-cooking ones.
• If you have trouble finding some of these ingredients in your local supermarket, look for them at a good health food shop.

nutrition per serve: Energy 1242 kJ (297 Cal); Fat 3.7 g; Saturated fat 0.6 g; Protein 6 g; Carbohydrate 59 g; Fibre 4.7 g; Cholesterol 0 mg; Sodium 10 mg

POACHED DRIED FRUIT WITH WHOLE SPICES

THIS FRUIT COMPOTE IS A LITTLE DIFFERENT FROM OTHER FRUIT COMPOTES WITH THE EXOTIC TOUCH OF ADDED SPICES.

1 orange
1 lemon
250 ml (9 fl oz/1 cup) unsweetened apple juice
6 whole cardamom pods, lightly crushed
6 whole cloves
1 cinnamon stick
375 g (13 oz) dried-fruit medley
3 tbsp soft brown sugar

PREP TIME: 10 MINUTES + 1 HOUR SOAKING
TOTAL COOKING TIME: 15 MINUTES
SERVES 8

Peel 3 large strips of orange rind, avoiding too much white pith. Peel the lemon rind into thick strips. Cut half the orange and lemon rinds into thin strips.

Put the apple juice, whole spices and thick strips of rind in a large saucepan with 750 ml (26 fl oz/3 cups) water and bring to the boil. Add the dried fruit. Remove from the heat and set aside for 1 hour.

Return to the heat, add the brown sugar and thin strips of rind and cover. Cook over low heat for 5 minutes, or until soft. Remove the fruit with a slotted spoon. Simmer the juice for another 5 minutes, or until reduced and thickened slightly. Serve the fruit warm or cold drizzled with juice.

HINT:
• This will keep well for at least a week covered and refrigerated.

nutrition per serve: Energy 630 kJ (150 Cal); Fat 0.2 g; Saturated fat 0 g; Protein 1.4 g; Carbohydrate 35 g; Fibre 3.7 g; Cholesterol 0 mg; Sodium 13 mg

THIS FLAVOURSOME AND
COLOURFUL FRUIT SALAD
CONTAINS AN ASSORTMENT
OF BERRIES, AND IS LADEN
WITH THE GOODNESS OF
VITAMINS, ANTIOXIDANTS
AND PHYTOCHEMICALS.

nutrition per serve: 500 kJ (119 Cal)
Fat 0.3 g
Saturated fat 0 g
Protein 1.9 g
Carbohydrate 24.9 g
Fibre 4.4 g
Cholesterol 0 mg
Sodium 6 mg

RED FRUIT SALAD WITH BERRIES

SYRUP
55 g (2 oz/¼ cup) caster (superfine) sugar
125 ml (4 fl oz/½ cup) unsweetened apple
and blackcurrant juice
1 star anise
1 tsp finely chopped lemon rind

250 g (9 oz/1⅔ cups) strawberries, hulled
and halved
155 g (5½ oz/1 cup) blueberries
155 g (5½ oz/1¼ cups) raspberries,
mulberries or other red berries

250 g (9 oz/1¼ cups) pitted cherries
5 small red plums, about 250 g (9 oz),
stones removed and quartered
low-fat yoghurt, to serve (optional)

PREP TIME: 5 MINUTES +
30 MINUTES COOLING +
30 MINUTES REFRIGERATION
TOTAL COOKING TIME: 5 MINUTES
SERVES 6

To make the syrup, put the sugar, juice, star anise, lemon rind and 125 ml (4 fl oz/½ cup) water in a small saucepan. Bring to the boil over medium heat, stirring to dissolve the sugar. Boil the syrup for 3 minutes, then set aside to cool for 30 minutes. When cool, strain the syrup.

Mix the fruit together in a large bowl and pour on the syrup. Mix well to coat the fruit in the syrup and refrigerate until cooled. Serve the fruit dressed with a little syrup and the yoghurt.

MUSHROOMS WITH SCRAMBLED EGGS AND WHOLEGRAIN BREAD

THIS IS A WHOLESOME, NOURISHING BREAKFAST, AND A GREAT WAY TO START THE DAY. IT PROVIDES GOOD AMOUNTS OF TOP-QUALITY PROTEIN, VITAMIN A, IRON AND FOLATE.

4 field mushrooms
olive oil spray
4 roma (plum) tomatoes, halved
3 tbsp balsamic vinegar
4 eggs, lightly beaten
4 egg whites, lightly beaten
3 tbsp low-fat milk

2 tbsp snipped fresh chives
8 thick slices wholegrain bread

PREP TIME: 15 MINUTES
COOKING TIME: 15 MINUTES
SERVES 4

Trim the mushroom stalks to 2 cm (¾ in) below the cap. Wipe the mushrooms with paper towels to remove any dirt and grit.

Spray both sides of the mushrooms with the oil and place on a non-stick baking tray with the tomatoes. Drizzle the mushrooms and tomatoes with the balsamic vinegar, then season with freshly ground black pepper and place under a medium grill (broiler) for 10–15 minutes, or until tender.

Meanwhile, put the eggs, egg whites, milk and chives in a bowl and whisk together to combine. Pour the mixture into a non-stick frying pan and cook over a low heat for 2–3 minutes, or until the egg begins to set, then gently stir with a wooden spoon to scramble.

Toast the wholegrain bread until golden brown, then cut on the diagonal. Serve with the mushrooms, tomato and scrambled eggs.

HINT:
• Use omega-3-enriched eggs instead of regular eggs to get more of the essential omega-3 fatty acids. Omega-3-enriched eggs are available in most large supermarkets and some health food shops.

nutrition per serve: Energy 1399 kJ (334 Cal); Fat 8.5 g; Saturated fat 2 g; Protein 20.8 g; Carbohydrate 39.5 g; Fibre 6.1 g; Cholesterol 188 mg; Sodium 572 mg

CORN CAKES WITH TOMATO SALSA

THESE TASTY CORN CAKES ARE A GREAT TREAT TO HAVE ON THE WEEKEND. THE TOMATO SALSA CONTAINS VITAMINS C AND E, AND BETA-CAROTENE.

TOMATO SALSA
2 tbsp diced red onion
2 firm tomatoes, seeded and diced
½ Lebanese (short) cucumber, seeded and diced
2 tbsp flat-leaf (Italian) parsley, chopped
1 tbsp olive oil
1 tbsp white vinegar

4 fresh corn cobs or 425 g (15 oz) tin corn kernels, drained
2 spring onions (scallions), finely chopped
2 eggs, lightly beaten
155 g (5½ oz/1¼ cups) self-raising flour
185 ml (6 fl oz/¾ cup) low-fat milk
olive oil spray

PREP TIME: 15 MINUTES
TOTAL COOKING TIME: 15 MINUTES
SERVES 4

To make the tomato salsa, put the red onion, tomato, cucumber and parsley in a bowl. Season with freshly ground black pepper, then add the oil and vinegar and toss together well to coat.

If using fresh corn, remove the kernels by cutting down the length of the cob with a sharp knife. Put the kernels in a small bowl with the spring onion and combine.

Whisk together the egg, self-raising flour and milk in a bowl until smooth. Fold in the corn and spring onion mixture and season to taste with freshly ground black pepper.

Heat a frying pan over medium heat and spray with oil. Working in batches, drop ¼ cup of batter per corn cake into the pan and allow enough space for spreading. Cook over medium heat for 2 minutes, or until golden. Turn over and cook for a further 1–2 minutes, or until golden. Repeat with the remaining batter to make 12 corn cakes.

To serve, stack three corn cakes on individual plates and top with some tomato salsa.

nutrition per serve: Energy 1442 kJ (345 Cal); Fat 9.4 g; Saturated fat 1.7 g; Protein 12.8 g; Carbohydrate 48.8 g; Fibre 5.4 g; Cholesterol 96 mg; Sodium 347 mg

BANANA BREAD WITH MAPLE RICOTTA

80 ml (2½ oz/⅓ cup) strong coffee
125 g (4½ oz/⅔ cup) soft brown sugar
1 egg
1 egg white
3 tbsp canola oil
1 tsp vanilla extract
3 ripe bananas, mashed
125 g (4½ oz/1 cup) plain flour
250 g (9 oz/2 cups) self-raising flour
½ tsp baking powder
1 tsp ground ginger

½ tsp ground nutmeg
1 tsp ground cinnamon
1 tsp bicarbonate of soda
200 g (7 oz) low-fat ricotta cheese
2 tbsp maple syrup
fresh berries, to serve

PREP TIME: 10 MINUTES

COOKING TIME: 55 MINUTES

MAKES 10–12 SLICES

Preheat the oven to 170°C (325°F/Gas 3). Lightly grease a 22 x 12 cm (8½ x 4½ in) loaf tin and line the base with baking paper. Heat the coffee in a small saucepan over low heat, add the brown sugar and stir until the sugar has dissolved.

Put the egg, egg white, oil and vanilla in a bowl and beat until just combined. Add the coffee mixture and banana.

Sift the flours, baking powder, ginger, nutmeg, cinnamon and bicarbonate of soda onto the mixture and stir gently to combine—do not overbeat. Spoon the mixture into the prepared loaf tin. Bake for 50 minutes, or until a skewer comes out clean when inserted into the centre. Leave in the tin for 10 minutes before turning out onto a wire rack to cool completely.

Combine the ricotta and maple syrup in a small bowl. Cut the banana bread into thick slices and serve with the maple ricotta and fresh berries.

HINT:
• Any left-over banana bread can be frozen in an airtight container with pieces of baking paper between each slice.

THIS REDUCED-FAT BANANA
BREAD IS A GREAT DISH TO SERVE
FOR BRUNCH. IT PROVIDES
CARBOHYDRATE, PROTEIN AND
MINERALS, AND THE MAPLE
RICOTTA AND BERRIES GIVE THE
ADDED BENEFIT OF CALCIUM,
FIBRE AND ANTIOXIDANTS.

nutrition per slice (12): Energy 1119 kJ (267 Cal)
Fat 6.4 g
Saturated fat 0.9 g
Protein 7.3 g
Carbohydrate 43.6 g
Fibre 3.6 g
Cholesterol 16 mg
Sodium 348 mg

OATY BUCKWHEAT PANCAKES

THESE DELICIOUS PANCAKES ARE ALSO NUTRITIOUS. THEY CONTAIN SLOWLY
DIGESTED CARBOHYDRATE, FIBRE AND PROTEIN, AND THE BERRIES ARE RICH
IN VITAMINS AND ANTIOXIDANTS.

BERRY SAUCE
55 g (2 oz/¼ cup) sugar
2 tsp lemon juice
250 g (9 oz/2 cups) raspberries

40 g (1½ oz/⅓ cup) buckwheat flour
100 g (3½ oz/⅔ cup) wholemeal
  (whole-wheat) flour
1½ tsp baking powder
25 g (1 oz/¼ cup) rolled (porridge) oats

1 egg yolk
375 ml (13 fl oz/1½ cups) buttermilk
3 egg whites
olive or canola oil spray
extra raspberries, to serve

PREP TIME: 15 MINUTES
COOKING TIME: 40 MINUTES
SERVES 4

To make the sauce, put the sugar, lemon juice and 60 ml (2 fl oz/¼ cup) water in a saucepan over medium heat and bring to the boil. Add the raspberries and cook over low heat for 3 minutes. Cool, then purée in a food processor or blender for 10 seconds.

Sift the flours into a bowl and return the husks to the bowl. Add the baking powder and rolled oats and combine. Make a well in the centre. Combine the egg yolk and buttermilk and add to the dry ingredients all at once. Stir to form a smooth batter. Whisk the egg whites until firm peaks form, then fold into the batter.

Heat a frying pan over medium heat and spray with oil. Pour 60 ml (2 fl oz/¼ cup) batter into the pan and swirl to form a 10 cm (4 in) circle. Cook for 1–2 minutes, or until bubbles appear on the surface. Turn and cook for 1–2 minutes, or until light brown. Transfer to a plate and keep warm. Repeat to make 8 pancakes. Serve with the berry sauce and raspberries.

nutrition per serve: Energy 1350 kJ (323 Cal); Fat 5.9 g; Saturated fat 2 g; Protein 13.3 g; Carbohydrate 49.5 g; Fibre 8 g; Cholesterol 53 mg; Sodium 368 mg

FRUIT FRAPPE

THIS DRINK IS A REFRESHING ANTIOXIDANT BREAKFAST COCKTAIL, RICH IN VITAMIN C, BETA-CAROTENE AND FIBRE. IT'S ALSO LOW IN SODIUM AND HIGH IN POTASSIUM, WHICH IS GOOD FOR BLOOD PRESSURE CONTROL.

10 dried apricot halves
205 g (7¼ oz/1½ cups) raspberries
1 banana, roughly chopped
1 mango, chopped
500 ml (17 fl oz/2 cups) orange juice
1 tbsp mint leaves
6 ice cubes

PREP TIME: 5 MINUTES + 10 MINUTES
  SOAKING
COOKING TIME: NIL
SERVES 4

Put the dried apricots in a heatproof bowl. Cover with 60 ml (2 fl oz/¼ cup) boiling water and soak for 10 minutes, or until plump. Drain, then roughly chop.

Put the chopped apricots, raspberries, banana, mango, orange juice, mint leaves and ice cubes in a blender, and blend until thick and smooth.

nutrition per serve: Energy 583 kJ (139 Cal); Fat 0.5 g; Saturated fat 0 g; Protein 2.6 g; Carbohydrate 28.1 g; Fibre 5.2 g; Cholesterol 0 mg; Sodium 13 mg

THE COMBINATION OF
RASPBERRIES AND BANANAS
MAKES THIS DRINK RICH IN
SOLUBLE FIBRE, WHICH CAN
HELP LOWER CHOLESTEROL
WHEN CONSUMED REGULARLY.

nutrition per serve: Energy 680 kJ (162 Cal)
Fat 0.6 g
Saturated fat 0.2 g
Protein 10.3 g
Carbohydrate 27 g
Fibre 3.2 g
Cholesterol 8 mg
Sodium 109 mg

LOW-FAT RASPBERRY AND BANANA SMOOTHIE

625 ml (21½ fl oz/2½ cups) skim milk
2 bananas
125 g (4½ oz/1 cup) raspberries
185 g (6½ oz/¾ cup) low-fat vanilla
   yoghurt
1 tbsp oat bran

PREP TIME: 5 MINUTES + 30 MINUTES
   CHILLING
COOKING TIME: NIL
SERVES 4

Put the milk in a covered container in the freezer for 30 minutes to make it very cold. It should be cold but not icy.

Peel and chop the bananas and put them in a blender. Add the raspberries, yoghurt, oat bran and 250 ml (9 fl oz/1 cup) of the milk. Blend for 30 seconds, or until smooth.

Add the remaining milk and blend for a further 30 seconds, or until combined. Pour into four glasses and serve immediately.

CARROT COCKTAIL

THIS DRINK IS AN EASY WAY TO BOOST YOUR NUTRIENT INTAKE AND TASTES MUCH BETTER THAN A VITAMIN SUPPLEMENT. IT IS RICH IN BETA-CAROTENE AND POTASSIUM, AND ALSO PROVIDES SOME FOLATE AND NIACIN.

10–12 carrots, quartered lengthways
125 ml (4 fl oz/½ cup) pineapple juice
125 ml (4 fl oz/½ cup) unsweetened
  orange juice
1–2 tsp honey, to taste
8 ice cubes

PREP TIME: 10 MINUTES
COOKING TIME: NIL
SERVES 2

Using the plunger, push the carrot pieces through a juicer.

Combine the carrot juice with the pineapple juice, orange juice, honey and ice cubes in a jug and serve.

nutrition per serve: Energy 714 kJ (171 Cal); Fat 0.5 g; Saturated fat 0 g; Protein 3.2 g; Carbohydrate 33.7 g; Fibre 8 g; Cholesterol 0 mg; Sodium 156 mg

PEACH AND ROCKMELON JUICE

A REFRESHING THIRST QUENCHER, THIS DRINK PROVIDES SWEET NATURAL SUGAR FOR ENERGY AND A BOOST OF VITAMIN C, BETA-CAROTENE, FOLATE, POTASSIUM AND FIBRE.

½ **rockmelon**

4 peaches

600 ml (21 fl oz) unsweetened orange juice

12 ice cubes

1 tbsp lime juice

PREP TIME: 10 MINUTES

COOKING TIME: NIL

SERVES 2

Peel the rockmelon, remove the seeds and roughly chop the flesh into bite-sized pieces. Cut a cross in the base of each peach. Put them in a heatproof bowl and cover with boiling water. Leave for 1–2 minutes, then remove with a slotted spoon, cool slightly and peel. Halve, remove the stone, and chop the flesh into bite-sized pieces.

Put the fruit in a blender with the orange juice and ice cubes, and blend until smooth. If the juice is too thick, add a little iced water. Stir in the lime juice and serve immediately.

nutrition per serve: Energy 984 kJ (235 Cal); Fat 0.8 g; Saturated fat 0 g; Protein 4.6 g; Carbohydrate 47.9 g; Fibre 5 g; Cholesterol 0 mg; Sodium 38 mg

SUMMER FRUIT SOY SMOOTHIE

1 banana

4 peaches, chopped

175 g (6 oz/¾ cup) apricot and mango soy
   yoghurt or vanilla soy yoghurt

1 tbsp oat bran

1 tsp natural vanilla extract

625 ml (21½ fl oz/2½ cups) reduced-fat
   plain soy milk or vanilla soy milk

1 tbsp maple syrup, optional

extra peach slices, to serve

ice cubes, to serve

PREP TIME: 10 MINUTES

COOKING TIME: NIL

SERVES 4

Put the banana, peach, yoghurt, oat bran, vanilla extract and 250 ml (9 fl oz/1 cup) of the soy milk in a blender and blend for 30 seconds, or until smooth.

Add the remaining soy milk and blend for a further 30 seconds, or until combined. Taste for sweetness and add the maple syrup, if using. Put the ice and extra peach slices in four glasses, pour in the smoothie and serve immediately.

THIS SOY SMOOTHIE IS LOW
IN CHOLESTEROL AND A GOOD
CHOICE FOR PEOPLE WHO
CAN'T TOLERATE DAIRY
PRODUCTS. USE CALCIUM-
ENRICHED SOY MILK FOR AN
EXTRA CALCIUM BOOST.

nutrition per serve: Energy 936 kJ (224 Cal)
Fat 1.9 g
Saturated fat 0.3 g
Protein 9.4 g
Carbohydrate 37.9 g
Fibre 4.5 g
Cholesterol 0 mg
Sodium 78 mg

SNACKS AND STARTERS

WHITE BEAN, CHICKPEA AND HERB DIP

THIS DELICIOUS DIP CONTAINS LESS FAT AND KILOJOULES THAN COMMERCIAL CREAM-BASED DIPS AND IS GREAT TO SNACK ON OR SERVE AT PARTIES AND BARBECUES. IT IS AN EASY WAY TO EAT MORE LEGUMES AND VEGETABLES.

3 slices wholegrain bread

3 tbsp low-fat milk

400 g (14 oz) tinned cannellini beans, drained and rinsed

300 g (10½ oz) tin chickpeas, drained and rinsed

2 spring onions (scallions), finely chopped

90 g (3¼ oz/⅓ cup) low-fat plain yoghurt

2 tbsp lemon juice

2 tsp finely grated lemon zest

1 tbsp chopped parsley

2 tsp chopped oregano

1 tbsp olive oil

vegetable crudités, to serve

PREP TIME: 10 MINUTES

COOKING TIME: NIL

SERVES 12

Remove the crusts from the bread, put the bread in a bowl and drizzle with the milk. Leave for 2 minutes, then mash with your fingertips until very soft.

Using a food processor or blender, process the cannellini beans, chickpeas, soaked bread, spring onion, yoghurt, lemon juice, zest, herbs and oil until combined but retaining some texture. Season well with freshly ground black pepper. Serve at room temperature with the vegetable crudités.

HINT:
• To make vegetable crudités, cut raw carrots, celery, zucchini (courgettes) and unpeeled Lebanese (short) cucumbers into 7 cm (2¾ in) sticks and raw cauliflower and broccoli into small florets.

nutrition per serve: Energy 314 kJ (75 Cal); Fat 2.2 g; Saturated fat 0.3 g; Protein 4 g; Carbohydrate 8.7 g; Fibre 2.7 g; Cholesterol 1 mg; Sodium 60 mg

PATE WITH TORTILLA CRISPS

WITH FAR LESS FAT THAN POTATO CHIPS AND REGULAR PÂTÉ, THIS SNACK IS A GOOD OPTION WHEN YOU'RE LOOKING FOR SOMETHING SAVOURY AND CRUNCHY TO NIBBLE ON.

1 tsp olive oil
1 small onion, chopped
2 garlic cloves, crushed
300 g (10½ oz) flat mushrooms, wiped
   clean and chopped
4 tbsp white wine or water
80 g (2¾ oz/1 cup) fresh wholemeal
   (whole-wheat) breadcrumbs
2 tbsp finely chopped thyme, plus extra to
   serve
2 tbsp chopped flat-leaf (Italian) parsley

1 tbsp lemon juice
4 large tortillas, about 20 cm (8 in) in
   diameter, each cut into 8 wedges
olive oil spray

PREP TIME: 15 MINUTES + 1 HOUR
   REFRIGERATION
COOKING TIME: 20 MINUTES
SERVES 4–6

Heat the oil in a large, deep frying pan. Add the onion and garlic and cook, stirring, for 2 minutes without browning. Add the mushrooms and wine. Cook, stirring for 1 minute, then cover and simmer for 5 minutes, stirring once or twice. Remove the lid and increase the heat to evaporate any liquid. Cool.

Put the mushroom mixture, breadcrumbs, herbs and lemon juice in a food processor or blender. Process until smooth and season well with freshly ground black pepper. Spoon into a serving bowl. Cover and refrigerate for at least 1 hour to allow the flavours to develop.

Preheat the oven to 180°C (350°F/Gas 4). Put the tortilla wedges on a large baking tray and lightly spray with the oil. Lightly sprinkle with freshly ground black pepper. Bake for 8 minutes, or until crisp. Serve the pâté with the tortilla crisps.

HINTS:
• Three slices of wholemeal (whole-wheat) bread, crusts removed, will yield about 1 cup of crumbs.
• Left-over tortilla crisps can be stored in the freezer for up to 1 month. Re-crisp them in a 170°C (325°F/Gas 3) oven for 5 minutes.

nutrition per serve (6): Energy 604 kJ (144 Cal); Fat 3.4 g; Saturated fat 0.5 g; Protein 5.5 g; Carbohydrate 18.8 g; Fibre 3.7 g; Cholesterol 0 mg; Sodium 181 mg

THIS TASTY DIP IS A GOOD WAY
TO INCLUDE LEGUMES IN YOUR
DIET. IT'S RELATIVELY LOW
IN KILOJOULES AND IS A RICH
SOURCE OF THE ANTIOXIDANT
BETA-CAROTENE.

nutrition per serve (8): Energy 384 kJ (92 Cal)
Fat 1.9 g
Saturated fat 0.3 g
Protein 5.4 g
Carbohydrate 11.9 g
Fibre 3.2 g
Cholesterol 1 mg
Sodium 164 mg

SWEET POTATO AND RED LENTIL DIP

2 tsp olive oil
1 small red onion, finely chopped
1 garlic clove, crushed
1 tsp grated fresh ginger
1 tbsp Thai red curry paste
200 g (7 oz) tinned reduced-salt
   diced tomatoes
125 g (4½ oz/½ cup) red lentils, drained
   and rinsed

375 ml (13 fl oz/1½ cups) reduced-salt
   chicken stock
250 g (9 oz) orange sweet potato,
   roughly chopped

PREP TIME: 20 MINUTES + COOLING TIME
COOKING TIME: 50 MINUTES
SERVES 6–8

Heat the oil in a saucepan over medium heat and cook the onion for 2 minutes, or until softened. Add the garlic, ginger and curry paste and stir for 30 seconds.

Add the tomatoes, lentils and stock to the pan. Bring to the boil, then reduce the heat to low, cover and simmer, stirring often, for 30 minutes, or until the mixture thickens and the lentils have softened but are still intact. Spoon the mixture into a bowl and refrigerate until cold.

Meanwhile, put the sweet potato in a steamer and cover with a lid. Sit the steamer over a wok or saucepan of boiling water and steam for 15 minutes, or until tender. Transfer to a bowl, cool and mash roughly with a fork.

Carefully stir the mashed sweet potato into the lentil mixture with a fork. Season to taste with freshly ground black pepper. Serve with pitta bread wedges, savoury crackers or crusty bread for dipping.

BEETROOT HUMMUS

THIS LOW-GI DIP CONTAINS GOOD AMOUNTS OF FIBRE, FOLATE, POTASSIUM AND PHYTOCHEMICAL ANTIOXIDANTS.

500 g (1 lb 2 oz) beetroot (beets), trimmed
1 tbsp olive oil
1 large onion, chopped
1 tbsp ground cumin
400 g (14 oz) tinned chickpeas, drained
　　and rinsed
1 tbsp tahini
90 g (3 ¼ oz/⅓ cup) low-fat plain yoghurt
3 garlic cloves, crushed

60 ml (2 fl oz/¼ cup) lemon juice
125 ml (4 fl oz/½ cup) reduced-salt
　　vegetable stock
Turkish bread, to serve (optional)

PREP TIME: 15 MINUTES
TOTAL COOKING TIME: 40 MINUTES
SERVES 8

Scrub the beetroot well. Bring a large saucepan of water to the boil and cook the beetroot for 40 minutes or until soft and cooked through. Drain and cool slightly before peeling.

Meanwhile, heat the oil in a frying pan over medium heat and cook the onion for 2 minutes, or until soft. Add the cumin and cook for a further 1 minute, or until fragrant.

Chop the beetroot and put in a food processor or blender with the onion mixture, chickpeas, tahini, yoghurt, garlic, lemon juice and stock and process until smooth and thoroughly combined. Spoon the hummus into a serving bowl and serve with Turkish bread.

HINTS:
• Beetroot hummus can be a great accompaniment to a main meal or is delicious as part of a meze platter with bruschetta or crusty bread. Its vivid colour sparks up any table.
• You can use 500 g (1 lb) of any vegetable to make the hummus. Try carrot or pumpkin.

nutrition per serve: Energy 487 kJ (116 Cal); Fat 4.8 g; Saturated fat 0.6 g; Protein 4.8 g; Carbohydrate 11.7 g; Fibre 4.1 g; Cholesterol <1 mg; Sodium 184 mg

TABOULEH WITH SOY GRITS

THIS TABOULEH IS A GOOD, GLUTEN-FREE ALTERNATIVE TO REGULAR
TABOULEH. IT IS LOW-GI AND A GOOD SOURCE OF FOLATE.

150 g (5½ oz) flat-leaf (Italian) parsley
180 g (6½ g/1 cup) soy grits
2 tbsp chopped mint
1 small red onion, cut into thin wedges
3 tomatoes, chopped
400 g (14 oz) tinned chickpeas, drained
   and rinsed
3 tbsp lemon juice

2 tbsp extra virgin olive oil
Lebanese or pitta bread, to serve (optional)
   (see Hints)

PREP TIME: 20 MINUTES + SOAKING
TOTAL COOKING TIME: NIL
SERVES 6–8

Remove all the parsley leaves from the stalks, roughly chop and put in a large
serving bowl.

Put the soy grits in a heatproof bowl and pour in 170 ml (5½ fl oz/⅔ cup) boiling water.
Leave to soak for 3 minutes, or until all the water has been absorbed.

Add the soy grits to the parsley, along with the mint, onion, tomato and chickpeas.
Drizzle with the lemon juice and olive oil. Season well with freshly ground black
pepper and toss together.

Serve with Lebanese or pitta bread.

HINTS:
• Soy grits are available from health food shops.
• For a complete gluten-free snack, serve with corn tortillas or gluten-free crackers.

nutrition per serve (8): Energy 938 kJ (224 Cal); Fat 12 g; Saturated fat 1.4 g; Protein 18.1 g;
Carbohydrate 9.5 g; Fibre 5.2 g; Cholesterol 0 mg; Sodium 93 mg

SMOKY EGGPLANT TAPENADE

1 large eggplant (aubergine), about 500 g
  (1 lb 2 oz)
310 g (11 oz/2 cups) pitted kalamata olives
5 anchovy fillets in brine, drained
35 g (1¼ oz/¼ cup) capers, rinsed and
  squeezed dry
3 garlic cloves, finely chopped
1 small handful flat-leaf (Italian) parsley
1 small handful basil

1 small handful oregano
1 tbsp lemon juice
1 tbsp extra virgin olive oil
crackers or vegetable crudités, to serve
  (optional)

PREP TIME: 20 MINUTES
COOKING TIME: 20 MINUTES
SERVES 10

Preheat the barbecue chargrill plate to high. Cook the eggplant, turning frequently, for 15–20 minutes, or until the skin is black all over and the flesh is soft. Remove from the heat. When cool enough to handle, cut off the stem, peel off the skin and roughly chop the eggplant flesh.

Put the olives, anchovies, capers, garlic, parsley, basil, oregano, lemon juice and oil in a small processor or blender. Process for 10–15 seconds, or until roughly chopped.

Add the chopped eggplant and blend in 3-second bursts for 15 seconds, or until the tapenade has a medium–smooth consistency with a little texture. Season with freshly ground black pepper and transfer to a serving bowl. Serve with crackers or vegetable crudités.

HINTS:
• Store in an airtight container in the refrigerator for up to a week.
• If you have a gas stove, you can put the eggplant directly on the open flame and follow the same cooking process as chargrilling. This will take half the time and give an even smokier flavour.

THIS TASTY TAPENADE MAKES
A GREAT DIP FOR PARTIES
OR A SNACK WITH VEGETABLE
CRUDITÉS OR CRACKERS. IT'S
ALSO DELICIOUS AS A SPREAD
ON BREAD INSTEAD OF
MARGARINE.

nutrition per serve: Energy 279 kJ (67 Cal)
Fat 2.5 g
Saturated fat 0.4 g
Protein 1.4 g
Carbohydrate 8.8 g
Fibre 1.9 g
Cholesterol 2 mg
Sodium 240 mg

SAN CHOY BAU

THIS TASTY CHINESE FAVOURITE IS GREAT TO SERVE AS A STARTER OR LIGHT MEAL WITH FRIENDS. IT'S IMPORTANT TO USE FRESH INGREDIENTS FOR THIS DISH TO ENJOY ITS CRISP, JUICY FLAVOURS.

4 dried Chinese mushrooms

3 tsp canola oil, for cooking

30 g (1 oz/¼ cup) slivered almonds, chopped

125 g (4 oz) water chestnuts, drained and finely chopped

1 carrot, finely chopped

4 spring onions (scallions), finely chopped

250 g (9 oz) lean minced (ground) pork

4 coriander (cilantro) roots, finely chopped

1 tbsp grated fresh ginger

12 lettuce leaves

hoisin sauce, to serve (optional)

SAUCE

1 tbsp reduced-sodium soy sauce

1 tbsp lime juice

1 tsp sesame oil

15 g (½ oz/¼ cup) chopped fresh coriander (cilantro) leaves

2 tbsp chopped fresh mint

PREP TIME: 25 MINUTES +
   10 MINUTES SOAKING

TOTAL COOKING TIME: 10 MINUTES

SERVES 4

Soak the mushrooms in a small bowl of hot water for 10 minutes, or until softened. Discard the tough stems and finely chop the mushroom caps.

To make the sauce, combine the soy sauce, lime juice, sesame oil, coriander and mint in a small jug.

Heat the wok until very hot, add 1 teaspoon of the oil and swirl around to coat the side. Add the almonds, water chestnuts, carrot and spring onion to the wok and stir-fry for 1 minute, or until they are lightly cooked but not browned—they should still be crisp. Remove from the wok and set aside.

Reheat the wok and add the remaining 2 teaspoons of canola oil. Stir-fry the minced pork, coriander root, ginger and mushrooms over medium–high heat for 2–3 minutes, or until the pork changes colour, but do not overcook the pork or it will be tough.

Add the sauce and stir to combine. Return the vegetable mixture to the wok and stir-fry for 1–2 minutes, or until heated through and the mixture is well combined. Spoon the pork mixture into the lettuce leaves and dollop with the hoisin sauce, to taste. Serve more hoisin sauce for dipping.

nutrition per serve: Energy 910 kJ (217 Cal); Fat 13.2 g; Saturated fat 1.8 g; Protein 16 g; Carbohydrate 7.5 g; Fibre 3.7 g; Cholesterol 19 mg; Sodium 253 mg

VIETNAMESE RICE PAPER ROLLS WITH DIPPING SAUCE

THESE FLAVOURSOME, REFRESHING RICE PAPER ROLLS ARE LOW IN FAT AND CHOLESTEROL-FREE. THEY ARE GREAT TO SERVE ON A HOT SUMMER DAY.

50 g (1¾ oz) dried rice vermicelli
200 g (7 oz) frozen soy beans
16 square (15 cm/6 in) rice paper wrappers
1 zucchini (courgette), julienned
1 Lebanese (short) cucumber, julienned
1 carrot, grated
20 g (¾ oz/1 cup) mint
100 g (3½ oz) firm tofu, cut into 1 cm (½ in) strips

DIPPING SAUCE
2 tbsp sweet chilli sauce
2 tbsp lime or lemon juice
2 tsp soft brown sugar
1 tsp reduced-sodium soy sauce or tamari
2 tbsp chopped coriander (cilantro) leaves

PREPARATION TIME: 40 MINUTES +
    5 MINUTES SOAKING
TOTAL COOKING TIME: 2 MINUTES
SERVES 4

Soak the vermicelli in hot water for 5 minutes, or until soft. Drain and cut into 5 cm (2 in) lengths with a pair of scissors. Bring a saucepan of water to the boil, add the soy beans and cook for 2 minutes. Drain well.

Working with no more than 2 rice paper wrappers at a time, dip each wrapper in a bowl of warm water for 10 seconds to soften. Drain, then lay out on a flat work surface.

Put a small amount of rice vermicelli on the bottom third of a wrapper, leaving a 2 cm (¾ in) border either side. Top with a little zucchini, cucumber, carrot, soy beans, mint and 2 strips of tofu. Keeping the filling compact and neat, fold in both sides and roll up tightly. Seal with a little water, if necessary. Cover with a damp cloth and repeat with the remaining rice paper wrappers and filling ingredients.

To make the dipping sauce, combine all the ingredients with 2 tablespoons water in a small bowl and stir together well. Serve with the rice paper rolls.

nutrition per serve: Energy 1315 kJ (314 Cal); Fat 5.7 g; Saturated fat 0.7 g; Protein 13.5 g; Carbohydrate 49.6 g; Fibre 4.5 g; Cholesterol 0 mg; Sodium 687 mg

SEAFOOD LOVERS WILL ENJOY THIS
LOW-GI DISH AS A SPECIAL TREAT.
THE PRAWNS PROVIDE IODINE,
PROTEIN AND THE BEANS ARE
RICH IN FIBRE.

nutrition per serve: Energy 1142 kJ (273 Cal)
Fat 7.4 g
Saturated fat 1.1 g
Protein 23.4 g
Carbohydrate 24.8 g
Fibre 8.3 g
Cholesterol 101 mg
Sodium 487 mg

ASIAN-STYLE PRAWNS WITH BEAN AND CORN SALAD

400 g (14 oz) tin cannellini beans, drained
   and rinsed
300 g (10½ oz) tin chickpeas, drained
   and rinsed
310 g (11 oz) tin corn kernels, drained
   and rinsed
1 tsp grated lime zest
2 tbsp chopped coriander (cilantro) leaves
500 g (1 lb 2 oz) raw large prawns (shrimp)
2 tbsp lemon juice

1 tbsp sesame oil
2 garlic cloves, crushed
2 tsp grated fresh ginger
olive or canola oil spray
lime quarters, to serve

PREP TIME: 10 MINUTES + 3 HOURS
   MARINATING
COOKING TIME: 5 MINUTES
SERVES 4

Combine the cannellini beans, chickpeas and corn kernels in a large bowl. Stir through the lime zest and coriander.

Peel the prawns, leaving the tails intact. Gently pull out the dark vein from each prawn back, starting at the head end.

To make the marinade, combine the lemon juice, sesame oil, garlic and ginger in a small bowl. Add the prawns and gently stir to coat them in the marinade. Cover and refrigerate for at least 3 hours.

Heat a barbecue hotplate until hot. Spray the hotplate with oil, then cook the prawns for 3–5 minutes, or until pink and cooked through. Brush frequently with marinade while cooking. Serve immediately with the bean mixture and wedges of lime.

HINT:
• Alternatively, the prawns can be threaded onto bamboo skewers. Soak the skewers in cold water for about 30 minutes. This will prevent the skewers burning during cooking. After marinating, thread the prawns evenly onto the skewers and cook as stated, turning and basting occasionally during cooking.

CHICKPEA FRITTERS

THESE FRITTERS ARE TASTY AND EASY TO EAT, AND WILL BE POPULAR WITH THE WHOLE FAMILY. THEY'RE AN EXCELLENT SOURCE OF FIBRE AND ARE FULL OF PROTEIN.

2 tsp olive or canola oil

4 spring onions (scallions), sliced

2 garlic cloves, finely chopped

1 small red chilli, seeded and finely chopped

2 x 300 g (10 oz) tins chickpeas, drained and rinsed

2 tbsp chopped coriander (cilantro) leaves

1 egg, lightly beaten

olive or canola oil spray

99% fat-free tomato salsa, to serve (optional)

100 g (3½ oz) mixed-leaf salad, to serve (optional)

PREP TIME: 20 MINUTES

COOKING TIME: 25 MINUTES

MAKES 6

Preheat the oven to 200°C (400°F/Gas 6). Line a baking tray with baking paper. Heat the oil in a large non-stick frying pan over medium heat. Add the spring onions, garlic and chilli and cook, stirring, for 1–2 minutes, or until the spring onion softens.

Put the chickpeas, spring onion mixture and coriander in a food processor or blender. Process until the mixture just starts to hold together. Do not overprocess—the mixture should be just roughly processed. Transfer to a bowl and mix in the egg. Using wet hands, shape the mixture into six even fritters.

Lightly spray the fritters with oil and put on prepared tray. Bake for 20 minutes turning once until lightly golden brown. Serve with salsa and a mixed-leaf salad.

nutrition per fritter: Energy 432 kJ (103 Cal); Fat 4.3 g; Saturated fat 0.7 g; Protein 5.5 g; Carbohydrate 9.1 g; Fibre 3.7 g; Cholesterol 31 mg; Sodium 168 mg

HERBED COTTAGE CHEESE POTATO

THIS NOURISHING LIGHT MEAL WILL KEEP YOU GOING. IT'S LOW IN FAT AND PROVIDES GOOD AMOUNTS OF B VITAMINS, BETA-CAROTENE, POTASSIUM AND PHOSPHORUS AS WELL AS CARBOHYDRATE.

4 large potatoes or orange sweet potatoes

200 g (7 oz) blanched, chopped spinach leaves (see Hint)

250 g (9 oz/1 cup) low-fat cottage cheese

2 tbsp chopped, mixed herbs (basil, parsley, oregano)

80 g (2¾ oz/½ cup) rinsed, chopped sun-dried tomatoes

125 g (4½ oz) diced mushrooms

PREP TIME: 20 MINUTES

COOKING TIME: 50 MINUTES

SERVES 4

Preheat the oven to 200°C (400°F/Gas 6). Bake the potatoes for 50 minutes, or until cooked through.

Put the spinach leaves, cottage cheese, herbs, sun-dried tomato and mushrooms in a bowl, and mix together well.

Make a deep cut along the top of each cooked sweet potato. Divide the topping among the baked potatoes. Serve hot.

HINT:
• To blanch the spinach, put the spinach leaves in a steamer over boiling water. Blanch for 1 minute then drain well.

nutrition per serve: Energy 1095 kJ (262 Cal); Fat 2.6 g; Saturated fat 0.6 g; Protein 18.9 g; Carbohydrate 33.9 g; Fibre 11.2 g; Cholesterol 7 mg; Sodium 164 mg

BAKED SWEET POTATOES WITH AVOCADO AND CORN SALSA

4 x 200 g (7 oz) orange sweet potatoes
1 red onion, finely chopped
1 avocado, finely chopped
1 tbsp lemon juice
130 g (4½ oz) tin corn kernels, drained
½ red capsicum (pepper), finely chopped

1 tbsp sweet chilli sauce
low-fat plain yoghurt, to serve

PREP TIME: 15 MINUTES
COOKING TIME: 50 MINUTES
SERVES 4

Preheat the oven to 200°C (400°F/Gas 6). Prick the sweet potatoes a few times with a skewer. Bake on an oven rack for 50 minutes, or until cooked through.

Meanwhile, put the onion, avocado, lemon juice, corn and capsicum in a bowl and mix together well. Stir in the chilli sauce and season to taste with freshly ground black pepper.

Make a deep cut along the top of each cooked sweet potato. Divide the topping among the sweet potatoes and add a dollop of low-fat plain yoghurt.

THIS VEGETARIAN BAKED SWEET
POTATO DISH IS A GREAT SOURCE
OF THE ANTIOXIDANTS LUTEIN,
BETA-CAROTENE AND ZEAXANTHIN.
IT'S ALSO LOW IN FAT.

nutrition per serve: Energy 1301 kJ (311 Cal)
Fat 13.5 g
Saturated fat 2.9 g
Protein 7.3 g
Carbohydrate 37.1 g
Fibre 5.5 g
Cholesterol 1 mg
Sodium 130 mg

SOUPS AND SALADS

JERUSALEM ARTICHOKE SOUP

JERUSALEM ARTICHOKES AREN'T REALLY ARTICHOKES AT ALL, BUT A TYPE OF TUBER. THEY ARE LOW IN KILOJOULES AND CHOLESTEROL-FREE AND HAVE A SLIGHTLY NUTTY FLAVOUR—DELICIOUS IN SOUPS.

1 tbsp olive oil
1 onion, roughly chopped
1 leek, white part only, chopped
1 celery stalk, chopped
2 garlic cloves, chopped
800 g (1 lb 12 oz) Jerusalem artichokes, cut into 5 cm (2 in) pieces
2 potatoes, about 250 g (9 oz), cut into 5 cm (2 in) pieces

1 tsp freshly grated nutmeg
250 ml (9 fl oz/1 cup) reduced-salt chicken stock or vegetable stock
500 ml (17 fl oz/2 cups) low-fat milk
2 tbsps finely snipped chives

PREP TIME: 20 MINUTES
COOKING TIME: 35 MINUTES
SERVES 4

Heat the oil in a large heavy-based saucepan over low heat. Add the onion, leek, celery and garlic and cook for 2 minutes. Cover and simmer, stirring occasionally, for 5 minutes. Do not allow the vegetables to brown.

Add the Jerusalem artichokes, potato and nutmeg and stir to combine. Cook for 2 minutes, then add the stock, 250 ml (9 fl oz/1 cup) water and 250 ml (9 fl oz/1 cup) of the milk. Bring to the boil, cover and cook for 20 minutes, or until the vegetables are tender.

Remove the saucepan from the heat. Set aside to cool slightly. Using a food processor or blender, process the soup for 10 seconds, or until roughly puréed. Season well with freshly ground black pepper. Stir in the remaining milk and half the chives and gently reheat the soup.

Ladle the soup into four bowls and sprinkle with the remaining chives and some freshly ground black pepper.

HINT:
• The Jerusalem artichokes can be replaced with an equal weight of potatoes. The soup will keep in the refrigerator, covered, for up to 4 days, or in an airtight container in the freezer for up to 1 month.

nutrition per serve: Energy 1255 kJ (300 Cal); Fat 5.5 g; Saturated fat 1 g; Protein 14 g; Carbohydrate 43.5 g; Fibre 9.2 g; Cholesterol 6 mg; Sodium 259 mg

SPLIT PEA SOUP

A GREAT WAY TO INCLUDE LEGUMES IN YOUR DIET, THIS NOURISHING SOUP IS LOW-FAT, LOW-GI AND HIGH IN FIBRE.

1 tbsp olive oil
1 large brown onion, chopped
1 large carrot, cut into 1 cm (½ in) cubes
1 large celery stalk, cut into 1 cm (½ in) cubes
2 bay leaves
1 tbsp finely chopped thyme
6 garlic cloves, finely chopped
440 g (15½ oz/2 cups) yellow split peas

1 litre (35 fl oz/4 cups) reduced-salt chicken stock
60 ml (2 fl oz/¼ cup) lemon juice
grainy bread, to serve (optional)
mixed-leaf salad, to serve (optional)

PREP TIME: 20 MINUTES
COOKING TIME: 1 HOUR 30 MINUTES
SERVES 6–8

Heat the oil in a large saucepan over medium heat. Add the onion, carrot and celery, and cook for 4–5 minutes, or until starting to brown. Add the bay leaves, thyme and garlic, and cook for 1 minute.

Stir in the split peas, then add the chicken stock and 1 litre (35 fl oz/4 cups) water. Cook for 1 hour 20 minutes, or until the split peas and vegetables are soft. Stir often during cooking to prevent the soup from sticking to the bottom of the pan, and skim any scum from the surface. Add a little extra water if the soup is too thick.

Remove the soup from the heat and discard the bay leaves. Stir in the lemon juice and season with freshly ground black pepper. Serve with grainy bread and a mixed-leaf salad.

nutrition per serve (8): Energy 941 kJ (225 Cal); Fat 3.6 g; Saturated fat 0.5 g; Protein 15.3 g; Carbohydrate 29.7 g; Fibre 6.9 g; Cholesterol 2 mg; Sodium 331 mg

NOTHING SOOTHES LIKE A
WARM BOWL OF SOUP ON
A COLD WINTER NIGHT. THIS
FRENCH CLASSIC IS SURE TO
MAKE YOU FEEL SATISFIED.

nutrition per serve: Energy 722 kJ (173 Cal)
Fat 8 g
Saturated fat 2.5 g
Protein 8.5 g
Carbohydrate 14.3 g
Fibre 4.5 g
Cholesterol 3 mg
Sodium 359 mg

ALSACE MUSHROOM SOUP

10 g (¼ oz) dried porcini mushrooms

1 tbsp olive oil

1 onion, roughly chopped

4 French shallots, chopped

1 large potato (about 185 g/6½ oz), chopped

1 celery stalk, chopped

2 garlic cloves, chopped

1 small red chilli, seeded and chopped

175 g (6 oz) flat mushrooms, roughly chopped

175 g (6 oz) Swiss brown mushrooms, roughly chopped

500 ml (17 fl oz/2 cups) reduced-salt chicken stock or vegetable stock

2 large thyme sprigs

1–2 tsp lemon juice, to taste

90 g (3¼ oz/⅓ cup) extra-light sour cream, to serve

2 tbsp finely chopped flat-leaf (Italian) parsley, to serve

1 tbsp grated lemon zest, to serve

PREP TIME: 25 MINUTES + 10 MINUTES SOAKING

COOKING TIME: 30 MINUTES

SERVES 4

Put the porcini mushrooms in a small bowl and pour 250 ml (9 fl oz/1 cup) hot water over them. Set aside to soften for 10 minutes.

Meanwhile, heat the oil in a large heavy-based saucepan. Add the onion, shallots, potato, celery, garlic and chilli. Stir for 2 minutes to coat the vegetables in the margarine. Reduce the heat, cover and simmer, stirring occasionally, for 5 minutes. Do not allow the vegetables to brown.

Add the fresh mushrooms to the saucepan and cook, stirring, for 2–3 minutes. Add the stock, 250 ml (9 fl oz/1 cup) water, thyme sprigs and porcini mushrooms with their soaking water. Slowly bring to the boil over low heat, then reduce the heat and simmer, covered, for 15 minutes. Discard the thyme sprigs. Set aside to cool slightly.

Using a food processor or blender, process the soup for 15–20 seconds, or until roughly puréed. The soup should still have texture. Add the lemon juice, to taste, and season well with freshly ground black pepper. Gently reheat the soup and ladle into warm bowls. Top with a spoonful of the sour cream and sprinkle with the parsley and lemon zest.

HINT:
• The soup will keep in the refrigerator, covered, for up to 4 days, or in an airtight container in the freezer for up to 1 month.

SCOTCH BROTH

BARLEY IS A GOOD GRAIN TO INCLUDE IN YOUR DIET IF YOU ARE TRYING TO LOWER YOUR CHOLESTEROL—IT'S LOW-GI AND A GOOD SOURCE OF SOLUBLE FIBRE. THIS BROTH ALSO CONTAINS B-GROUP VITAMINS, IRON AND ZINC.

1 kg (2 lb 4 oz) lamb shanks, cut in half
   through the bone (ask your butcher
   to do this)
3 onions, chopped
3 turnips, chopped
2 carrots, chopped
1 tbsp black peppercorns
110 g (3¾ oz/½ cup) pearl barley
1 carrot, diced, extra
2 onions, finely chopped, extra

2 turnips, diced, extra
1 leek, white part only, chopped
1 celery stalk, diced
chopped flat-leaf (Italian) parsley,
   to serve

PREP TIME: 40 MINUTES + 1 HOUR SOAKING +
   OVERNIGHT REFRIGERATION
COOKING TIME: 3 HOURS 35 MINUTES
SERVES 8

To make the stock, put the lamb shanks, onion, turnip, carrot, peppercorns and 2 litres (70 fl oz/8 cups) water in a large saucepan. Bring to the boil, reduce the heat and simmer, covered, for 3 hours. Skim the surface as required.

Remove the shanks and any meat that has fallen off the bones and cool slightly. Remove the meat from the bones and finely chop, then cover and refrigerate. Strain the stock, discarding the vegetables. Cool the stock and refrigerate overnight, or until the fat has set on top and can be spooned off. Cover the barley with water and soak for 1 hour, then drain.

Put the stock in a large pan and gently reheat. Add the barley, extra carrot, onion and turnip, and the leek and celery. Bring to the boil, reduce the heat and simmer for 30 minutes, or until the barley and vegetables are just cooked. Return the meat to the pan and simmer for 5 minutes. Season well with freshly ground black pepper and serve with the parsley.

nutrition per serve: Energy 952 kJ (228 Cal); Fat 6.7 g; Saturated fat 3.3 g; Protein 22.5 g; Carbohydrate 16.3 g; Fibre 5.7 g; Cholesterol 65 mg; Sodium 91 mg

BEETROOT AND RED CAPSICUM SOUP

THIS COLOURFUL SOUP WITH THE GOODNESS OF BEETROOT AND CAPSICUM IS LOW IN FAT AND A RICH SOURCE OF THE ANTIOXIDANT BETA-CAROTENE.

6 beetroot (beets), about 600 g (1 lb 5 oz)
   without stems and leaves
1 tbsp olive oil
1 red onion, chopped
1 celery stalk, chopped
1 garlic clove, chopped
1 large red capsicum (pepper), chopped
410 g (14½ oz) tin reduced-salt diced
   tomatoes
1 tbsp red wine vinegar

extra-light sour cream or low-fat plain
   yoghurt, to serve (optional)
2 tbsp finely snipped chives, to serve

PREP TIME: 20 MINUTES
COOKING TIME: 50 MINUTES
SERVES 4

Peel the beetroot with a vegetable peeler and cut it into 3 cm (1¼ in) cubes. Put the beetroot in a large saucepan with 1 litre (35 fl oz/4 cups) water. Slowly bring to the boil over low–medium heat, then reduce the heat and simmer for 25–30 minutes, or until the beetroot is tender when pierced with a fork. Remove about ½ cup of beetroot cubes, dice finely and set aside.

Meanwhile, heat the oil in a large heavy-based saucepan over medium heat. Add the onion, celery, garlic and capsicum and stir to coat the vegetables in the oil. Reduce the heat to low, cover and cook, stirring occasionally, for 10 minutes. Do not allow the vegetables to brown. Add the chopped tomatoes and vinegar and simmer for 10 minutes.

Transfer the tomato mixture to the saucepan containing the beetroot and remove the pan from the heat. Set aside to cool slightly. Using a food processor or blender, process the soup for 20–30 seconds, or until smooth. Season well with freshly ground black pepper.

Ladle the soup into four warm bowls and top with a spoonful of sour cream, the reserved diced beetroot and the chives.

HINT:
• The soup will keep in the refrigerator, covered, for up to 4 days, or in an airtight container in the freezer for up to 1 month.

nutrition per serve: Energy 603 kJ (144 Cal); Fat 5 g; Saturated fat 0.6 g; Protein 4.3 g; Carbohydrate 17.4 g; Fibre 5.5 g; Cholesterol 0 mg; Sodium 99 mg

SPICED PUMPKIN AND LENTIL SOUP

1 tbsp olive oil
1 large onion, chopped
3 garlic cloves, chopped
1 tsp ground turmeric
½ tsp ground coriander
½ tsp ground cumin
½ tsp chilli flakes
700 g (1 lb 9 oz/4½ cups) pumpkin
  (winter squash), chopped

125 g (4½ oz/½ cup) tinned red lentils,
  drained and rinsed
90 g (3¼ oz/⅓ cup) plain low-fat yoghurt,
  to serve

PREP TIME: 20 MINUTES
COOKING TIME: 30 MINUTES
SERVES 4

Heat the oil in a large saucepan over medium heat. Add the onion and garlic and fry for 5 minutes, or until softened, being careful not to burn the garlic. Add the turmeric, coriander, cumin and chilli flakes and fry, stirring constantly, for 2 minutes.

Add the pumpkin, red lentils and 1 litre (35 fl oz/4 cups) boiling water. Bring to the boil, then reduce the heat and simmer, covered, for 20 minutes, or until the pumpkin and lentils are tender. Set aside to cool for 5 minutes.

Using a food processor or blender, process the soup for 25–35 seconds, or until evenly chopped. Season well with freshly ground black pepper and reheat the soup.

Ladle the soup into four bowls, top with a spoonful of the yoghurt and sprinkle with more pepper.

THIS IS A NUTRITIOUS AND
SATISFYING SOUP THAT IS SURE
TO MAKE YOU FEEL FULL.
THE ADDITION OF LENTILS
MAKES IT MORE NUTRITIOUS
AND LOWER GI THAN REGULAR
PUMPKIN SOUP.

nutrition per serve: Energy 977 kJ (233 Cal)
Fat 6.2 g
Saturated fat 1.3 g
Protein 13.5 g
Carbohydrate 27.6 g
Fibre 7.7 g
Cholesterol 1 mg
Sodium 28 mg

COUSCOUS SALAD

THIS SALAD IS A GOOD CHOICE FOR ACTIVE PEOPLE. IT'S LOW IN FAT AND HIGH IN CARBOHYDRATE AND PROVIDES GOOD AMOUNTS OF FIBRE, BETA-CAROTENE AND B-GROUP VITAMINS.

300 g (10½ oz) orange sweet potato, cubed
100 g (3½ oz) green beans, halved
350 g (12 oz/2 cups) instant couscous
500 ml (17 fl oz/2 cups) boiling reduced-salt chicken stock
200 g (7 oz) cherry tomatoes, halved
150 g (5½ oz/1 cup) frozen corn kernels, thawed
155 g (5½ oz/1 cup) frozen peas, thawed
1 red capsicum (pepper), chopped
60 g (2¼ oz/1 cup) chopped parsley
25 g (1 oz/½ cup) chopped mint

DRESSING
1 garlic clove, crushed
2 tbsp lemon juice
1 tbsp olive oil
1 tsp honey
½ tsp grainy mustard

PREP TIME: 20 MINUTES + 5 MINUTES STANDING
COOKING TIME: 15 MINUTES
SERVES 6

Boil or steam the sweet potato and beans in separate saucepans until tender, then drain. Put the couscous in a large bowl and pour on the boiling stock. Cover and leave for 5 minutes, or until all the liquid has been absorbed. Fluff with a fork to separate the grains.

Add the sweet potato, beans, tomato, corn, peas, capsicum and herbs to the couscous, and mix together well.

Put the garlic, lemon juice, oil, honey and mustard in a bowl, and whisk together. Pour the dressing over the salad and toss well.

nutrition per serve: Energy 1487 kJ (355 Cal); Fat 4.1 g; Saturated fat 0.6 g; Protein 13.3 g; Carbohydrate 62.4 g; Fibre 5.9 g; Cholesterol 2 mg; Sodium 234 mg

CHICKPEA AND ROAST VEGETABLE SALAD

THIS HEALTHY SALAD IS AN EASY WAY TO EAT LEGUMES AND VEGETABLES. IT IS LOW IN FAT AND RICH IN BETA-CAROTENE AND SOLUBLE FIBRE.

500 g (1 lb 2 oz) butternut pumpkin, cubed
2 red capsicums (peppers), halved
4 slender eggplants (aubergines), cut in
    half lengthways
4 zucchini (courgettes), cut in half
    lengthways
4 onions, quartered
olive oil spray
2 x 300 g (10 oz) tins chickpeas, drained
    and rinsed
2 tbsp chopped fresh flat-leaf (Italian)
    parsley

DRESSING
3 tbsp lemon juice
2 tbsp olive oil
1 garlic clove, crushed
1 tsp finely chopped thyme

PREP TIME: 25 MINUTES +
    30 MINUTES STANDING
TOTAL COOKING TIME: 40 MINUTES
SERVES 8

Preheat the oven to 220°C (425°F/Gas 7). Line 2 baking trays with baking paper and lay out the vegetables in a single layer and spray them with oil.

Bake for 40 minutes, or until the vegetables are tender and begin to brown slightly on the edges. Cool. Remove the skins from the capsicum if you want. Chop the capsicum, eggplant and zucchini into pieces, then put the vegetables in a bowl with the chickpeas and half the parsley.

Whisk together all the dressing ingredients. Season with freshly ground black pepper, then toss with the vegetables. Leave for 30 minutes, then sprinkle with the rest of the parsley.

nutrition per serve: Energy 661 kJ (158 Cal); Fat 6.8 g; Saturated fat 1.1 g; Protein 6.2 g; Carbohydrate 15.6 g; Fibre 5.3 g; Cholesterol 0 mg; Sodium 122 mg

THIS LOW-GI SALAD IS QUICK AND EASY TO PREPARE FOR LUNCH OR DINNER. IT CONTAINS SOME ESSENTIAL OMEGA-3 FATTY ACIDS AND GOOD AMOUNTS OF POTASSIUM, ANTIOXIDANTS, FOLATE AND PHOSPHORUS.

nutrition per serve (6): Energy 1358 kJ (324 Cal)
Fat 5.5 g
Saturated fat 0.9 g
Protein 16 g
Carbohydrate 50.1 g
Fibre 3.7 g
Cholesterol 16 mg
Sodium 574 mg

HERBED PASTA AND SALMON SALAD

400 g (14 oz) small pasta shells
250 g (9 oz) cherry tomatoes, quartered,
    or halved, if small
1 large yellow capsicum (pepper), seeded
    and diced
2 celery stalks, thinly sliced
3 spring onions (scallions), thinly sliced
40 g (1½ oz/¼ cup) pitted green olives
    in brine, drained and chopped
2 tbsp capers, rinsed and chopped
    (optional)
200 g (7 oz) smoked salmon, sliced
1 handful basil, finely shredded
3 tbsp finely chopped flat-leaf (Italian)
    parsley

DRESSING
1 tbsp olive oil
1½ tbsps white wine vinegar
½ tsp dijon mustard
1 tsp honey

PREP TIME: 15 MINUTES
COOKING TIME: 10 MINUTES
SERVES 4–6

Cook the pasta in a large saucepan of boiling water for 10 minutes, or until *al dente*. Rinse under cold water to cool. Drain. Put in a large bowl.

To make the dressing, whisk all the ingredients together. Put all the other ingredients into the bowl with the pasta, add the dressing and toss together. Season with freshly ground black pepper and serve.

HINT:
• Any type of small pasta shapes can be used in this recipe.

81

TUNA AND BEAN SALAD

BASED ON FISH AND BEANS, THIS SALAD CONTAINS FILLING PROTEIN, LOW-GI
CARBOHYDRATE AND FIBRE, PLUS GOOD AMOUNTS OF B-GROUP VITAMINS,
VITAMIN C, POTASSIUM AND HEART-HEALTHY OMEGA-3 FATTY ACIDS.

100 g (3½ oz) green beans, chopped
400 g (14 oz) tin butterbeans (lima beans),
   drained and rinsed
425 g (15 oz) tin tuna in spring water,
   drained
200 g (7 oz) cherry tomatoes, quartered
1 red onion, thinly sliced
100 g (3½ oz) mixed salad leaves
100 g (3½ oz) baby rocket (arugula) leaves

DRESSING
1 tbsp extra virgin olive oil
2 tbsp lemon juice
1 tsp honey
1 garlic clove, crushed
2 tbsp chopped dill

PREP TIME: 20 MINUTES + 10 MINUTES
   REFRIGERATION
COOKING TIME: 5 MINUTES
SERVES 4

Steam the green beans until tender, rinse under cold water and drain. Put the green
and butterbeans, tuna, tomato and onion in a bowl, and toss well.

To make the dressing, whisk all the ingredients together. Pour the dressing over the
tuna mixture, cover and refrigerate for 10 minutes.

Combine the salad leaves and rocket, and arrange on a salad platter. Top with the tuna
mixture and serve.

nutrition per serve: Energy 984 kJ (235 Cal); Fat 7.1 g; Saturated fat 1.4 g; Protein 25.6 g;
Carbohydrate 14.1 g; Fibre 7 g; Cholesterol 39 mg; Sodium 85 mg

COLD CHICKEN AND MANGO SALAD WITH HONEY DRESSING

THIS TANGY SALAD IS BURSTING WITH FLAVOUR. IT IS VERY EASY TO MAKE, COMPLETELY SATISFYING AND LOW IN FAT.

DRESSING
2 tbsp rice vinegar
3 tsp honey
3 cm (1¼ in) piece ginger, chopped
1 tbsp canola oil
1 tsp sesame oil

125 g (4½ oz) mixed Asian salad leaves
1 large mango, thinly sliced
125 g (4½ oz/1 cup) yellow or red cherry
   tomatoes, halved

½ small red onion, sliced into thin wedges
1 cold barbecued chicken, fat and skin
   removed, meat shredded
30 g (1 oz/¾ cup) snow pea (mangetout)
   sprouts, trimmed
2 tsp toasted sesame seeds

PREP TIME: 15 MINUTES
COOKING TIME: NIL
SERVES 4

To make the dressing, put the vinegar, honey and ginger in a mini food processor or blender and process in 3-second bursts for 20 seconds, or until finely chopped. With the motor running, slowly pour in the oils and blend for 20 seconds, or until thick and creamy.

Arrange the salad leaves on individual plates and top with the mango, tomatoes, onion, chicken and snow pea sprouts. Drizzle with the dressing and sprinkle with the sesame seeds. Serve immediately.

nutrition per serve: Energy 1475 kJ (352 Cal); Fat 16.7 g; Saturated fat 3.4 g; Protein 33.4 g; Carbohydrate 15.9 g; Fibre 2.5 g; Cholesterol 114 mg; Sodium 115 mg

PESTO BEEF SALAD

1 large red capsicum (pepper)
1 large yellow capsicum (pepper)
olive or canola oil spray
100 g (3½ oz) lean beef fillet steak,
  trimmed
125 g (4½ oz) penne
100 g (3½oz) button mushrooms,
  quartered

PESTO
½ bunch basil (about 50 g/1¾ oz leaves)
2 garlic cloves, chopped
2 tbsp pepitas (pumpkin seeds)
1 tbsp olive oil
2 tbsp orange juice
1 tbsp lemon juice

PREP TIME: 30 MINUTES + 5 MINUTES
  STANDING
COOKING TIME: 25 MINUTES
SERVES 4

Cut the capsicums into large flat pieces, removing the seeds and membrane. Put, skin side up, under a hot grill (broiler) until blackened. Leave covered with a tea towel (dish towel) until cool, then peel away the skin and chop the flesh.

Heat a frying pan over medium heat and spray with oil, then cook the steak over high heat for 3–4 minutes on each side. Remove and leave for 5 minutes before cutting into thin slices.

To make the pesto, finely chop the basil, garlic and pepitas in a food processor. With the motor running, add the oil, orange and lemon juice. Season well with freshly ground black pepper.

Meanwhile, cook the pasta in a large saucepan of boiling water for 10 minutes, or until *al dente*. Drain well and toss with the pesto in a large bowl.

Add the capsicum pieces, steak slices and mushroom quarters to the penne and toss to distribute evenly. Serve immediately.

THIS TASTY LOW-GI PASTA SALAD IS A GREAT CHOICE FOR PEOPLE WHO NEED TO EAT MORE IRON. THE PESTO IN THIS DISH IS MUCH LOWER IN FAT THAN REGULAR PESTO, AND THE DISH PROVIDES GOOD AMOUNTS OF ANTIOXIDANTS, VITAMIN C AND BETA-CAROTENE.

nutrition per serve: Energy 1028 kJ (246 Cal)
Fat 9.5 g
Saturated fat 1.7 g
Protein 12.3 g
Carbohydrate 25.7 g
Fibre 3.6 g
Cholesterol 17 mg
Sodium 20 mg

TANDOORI LAMB SALAD

THIS INDIAN-STYLE SALAD IS HIGH IN PROTEIN AND A GOOD SOURCE OF IRON, ZINC, POTASSIUM, PHOSPHORUS, FOLATE, NIACIN AND BETA-CAROTENE.

250 g (9 oz/1 cup) low-fat plain yoghurt
2 garlic cloves, crushed
2 tsp grated fresh ginger
2 tsp ground turmeric
2 tsp ground garam masala
¼ tsp paprika
2 tsp ground coriander
500 g (1 lb 2 oz) lean lamb fillets
4 tbsp lemon juice
1½ tsp chopped coriander leaves

1 tsp chopped mint
150 g (5 oz) mixed salad leaves
1 large mango, cut into strips
2 Lebanese (short) cucumbers, julienned

PREP TIME: 20 MINUTES + OVERNIGHT
MARINATING
TOTAL COOKING TIME: 15 MINUTES
SERVES 4

Mix the yoghurt, garlic, ginger, dried herbs and spices in a bowl, add a little food colouring (if using) and toss with the lamb to thoroughly coat. Cover and refrigerate overnight.

Grill (broil) the lamb on a foil-lined baking tray under high heat for 7 minutes each side, or until the marinade starts to brown. Set aside for 5 minutes before serving.

Mix the lemon juice, coriander and mint then season with freshly ground black pepper. Toss with the salad leaves, mango and cucumber, then arrange on plates. Slice the lamb and serve over the salad.

nutrition per serve: Energy 1021 kJ (244 Cal); Fat 5.4 g; Saturated fat 2.1 g; Protein 31.4 g; Carbohydrate 14.5 g; Fibre 3.5 g; Cholesterol 84 mg; Sodium 144 mg

VIETNAMESE RICE NOODLE SALAD

THIS FRESH, ZESTY VIETNAMESE CLASSIC IS A GOOD CHOICE ON A HOT
SUMMER DAY. IT PROVIDES ANTIOXIDANTS AND MINERALS.

200 g (7 oz) dried vermicelli
80 g (3 oz/½ cup) crushed roasted peanuts
10 g (¼ oz/½ cup) Vietnamese mint, torn
15 g (½ oz/½ cup) coriander (cilantro)
  leaves
½ red onion, cut into thin wedges
1 green mango, julienned
1 Lebanese (short) cucumber, halved
  lengthways and thinly sliced on
  the diagonal

LEMON GRASS DRESSING
125 ml (4 fl oz/½ cup) lime juice
1 tbsp shaved palm sugar or brown sugar
3 tbsp seasoned rice vinegar
2 lemon grass stems, finely chopped
3 makrut (kaffir lime) leaves, finely
  shredded

PREP TIME: 20 MINUTES + 10 MINUTES
  STANDING + 30 MINUTES REFRIGERATION
TOTAL COOKING TIME: NIL
SERVES 4–6

Put the rice vermicelli in a bowl and cover with boiling water. Leave for 10 minutes or until soft, then drain, rinse under cold water and cut into short lengths.

Put the vermicelli, peanuts, mint, coriander, onion, mango and cucumber in a large bowl and toss together.

To make the dressing, put all the ingredients in a jar with a lid and shake.

Toss the salad and dressing and refrigerate for 30 minutes before serving.

nutrition per serve (6): Energy 988 kJ (236 Cal); Fat 6.7 g; Saturated fat 0.8 g; Protein 6.8 g; Carbohydrate 35.5 g; Fibre 2.6 g; Cholesterol 0 mg; Sodium 9 mg

ADDING A VARIETY OF HEALTHY
INGREDIENTS FROM DIFFERENT
FOOD GROUPS MAKES A SALAD
MORE SATISFYING AND NUTRITIOUS,
AND HELPS YOU MEET HEALTHY
EATING GUIDELINES. THIS SALAD
FITS THE BILL!

nutrition per serve: Energy 989 kJ (236 Cal)
Fat 7.7 g
Saturated fat 2 g
Protein 23.9 g
Carbohydrate 15.7 g
Fibre 3.7 g
Cholesterol 76 mg
Sodium 150 mg

CHICKEN AND SWEET POTATO SALAD

4 roma (plum) tomatoes, quartered
   lengthways
300 g (10½ oz) eggplant (aubergine),
   quartered lengthways
olive oil spray
500 g (1 lb 2 oz) orange sweet potato,
   cut into 2 cm (¾ in) slices
1 large red onion, sliced into thin wedges

1 barbecued chicken
2 tbsp chopped coriander (cilantro) leaves
2–3 tbsp balsamic vinegar
2 handfuls rocket (arugula)

PREP TIME: 30 MINUTES

COOKING TIME: 50 MINUTES

SERVES 6

Preheat the oven to 200°C (400°F/Gas 6). Put the tomatoes and eggplant on a large, non-stick baking tray, spray with a little oil and season with freshly ground black pepper. Bake, turning the eggplant halfway through, for 25–30 minutes.

Meanwhile, steam the sweet potato for 15 minutes, or until just tender. Put in a large bowl with the tomato and eggplant.

Lightly spray a small non-stick frying pan with oil, add the onion and cook over a low heat for 6 minutes, or until golden. Set aside.

Remove the skin and bones from the chicken and discard. Cut the chicken meat into bite-sized pieces and add to the vegetables with the coriander and 1 tablespoon balsamic vinegar. Toss gently.

Put the rocket on a platter, then the chicken mixture and top with the onion. Drizzle with the remaining balsamic vinegar to taste. Serve with thick slices of wholegrain bread.

HINT:
• You can substitute the barbecued chicken with freshly cooked chicken breast fillets or you can use precooked chicken breast meat, which you'll find in the freezer section of the supermarket.

MAIN MEALS

CHICKEN CACCIATORE

THIS LOW-FAT VERSION OF A POPULAR ITALIAN DISH PROVIDES PROTEIN, MONOUNSATURATED FAT, POTASSIUM, NIACIN AND ANTIOXIDANTS.

500 g (1 lb 2 oz) lean chicken breast fillets
plain (all-purpose) flour, for dusting
2 tsp olive oil
2 onions, thinly sliced
2 garlic cloves, finely chopped
2 anchovy fillets in brine, drained and
  chopped
440 g (15½ oz) tin reduced-salt diced
  tomatoes
125 ml (4 fl oz/½ cup) dry white wine
3 tbsp no-added-salt tomato paste
  (concentrated purée)

1 tsp soft brown sugar
6 Kalamata olives, pitted and chopped
chopped fresh flat-leaf (Italian) parsley,
  to garnish
fusilli pasta or boiled potatoes, to serve
  (optional)

PREP TIME: 25 MINUTES
COOKING TIME: 40 MINUTES
SERVES 4

Trim any fat from the chicken and lightly dust the chicken in plain flour. Heat the oil in a large, heavy-based non-stick frying pan and cook the chicken over high heat for 10 minutes, turning until golden and almost cooked. (If the chicken begins to stick, sprinkle with water and reduce the heat.) Remove, drain on paper towels, cover and set aside.

Add the onion to the pan with the garlic, anchovies and 1 tablespoon water. Cover and cook for 5 minutes, stirring. Add the tomato, wine, tomato paste, sugar and 200 ml (7 fl oz) water. Bring to the boil, then reduce the heat and simmer for 20 minutes. Season with freshly ground black pepper.

Return the chicken and juices to the pan. Add the olives and simmer for 5 minutes, or until the chicken is heated through. Garnish with parsley. Serve with fusilli pasta or boiled potatoes.

nutrition per serve: Energy 1063 kJ (254 Cal); Fat 4.5 g; Saturated fat 1.1 g; Protein 30.8 g; Carbohydrate 15.2 g; Fibre 3.3 g; Cholesterol 83 mg; Sodium 203 mg

CORAL TROUT WITH GARLIC TOMATOES AND GREMOLATA

STRONG FLAVOURS ABOUND IN THIS TASTY, LOW-FAT DISH. IT IS QUICK TO PREPARE AND IS A GOOD SOURCE OF PROTEIN, BETA-CAROTENE AND OTHER ANTIOXIDANTS.

8 vine-ripened tomatoes, halved

12 garlic cloves, unpeeled

2 tbsp balsamic vinegar

1 tbsp soft brown sugar

olive or canola oil spray

750 g (1 lb 10 oz) new potatoes

300 g (10½ oz) asparagus, trimmed

4 x 200 g (7 oz) coral trout fillets or firm
   white fish fillets

GREMOLATA

3 handfuls flat-leaf (Italian) parsley, finely
   chopped

2 tsp lemon zest

2 garlic cloves, finely chopped

PREP TIME: 20 MINUTES

COOKING TIME: 55 MINUTES

SERVES 4

Preheat the oven to 200°C (400°F/Gas 6). Line a large baking tray with baking paper. Put the tomatoes, cut-side-up, on the prepared tray. Scatter around the garlic cloves. Pour over the combined balsamic vinegar and sugar. Spray lightly with the oil. Bake the tomatoes and garlic for 30 minutes, or until softened. Remove the garlic after 15 minutes and baste the tomatoes with the balsamic vinegar and sugar. Squeeze out the soft garlic from the cloves and add to the mushy tomatoes.

Combine the gremolata ingredients in a small bowl.

Bring a large saucepan of water to the boil. Cook the potatoes for 12 minutes, or until cooked when tested with a skewer. Drain. Steam the asparagus for 3–4 minutes, or until just tender.

Pat the fish dry with paper towels. Spray a large, non-stick frying pan with oil and lightly spray the fish. Cook the fish for 3–4 minutes on each side, or until browned on both sides and just cooked through.

To serve, pile the tomato and garlic onto serving plates. Top with the fish fillets and spoon over some gremolata. Serve with the boiled new potatoes and steamed asparagus to the side.

nutrition per serve: Energy 1757 kJ (420 Cal); Fat 5.3 g; Saturated fat 1.3 g; Protein 48.7 g; Carbohydrate 36.3 g; Fibre 10.9 g; Cholesterol 96 mg; Sodium 169 mg

BLUE-EYE COD IN CHERMOULA

CHERMOULA
1½ tbsp cumin seeds
2 tsp coriander seeds
1 tbsp sweet paprika
pinch cayenne pepper
2 large handfuls coriander (cilantro),
    chopped
1 large handful flat-leaf (Italian) parsley,
    chopped
4 large garlic cloves, crushed
2 tbsp olive oil
4 tbsp lemon juice

4 x 150 g (5½ oz) blue-eye cod steaks or
    other firm white fish steaks
700 g (1 lb 9 oz) small new potatoes
500 g (1 lb 2 oz) zucchini (courgette),
    thickly sliced
115 g (4 oz) fresh baby corn

PREP TIME: 20 MINUTES + 1 HOUR
    MARINATING
COOKING TIME: 20 MINUTES
SERVES 4

To make the chermoula, place the cumin and coriander seeds, paprika and cayenne pepper in a small, dry frying pan and toast for 1 minute over a medium heat, or until fragrant. Put in a spice grinder, or use a mortar and pestle, and grind to a fine powder. Put in a food processor with the coriander, parsley, garlic, oil and lemon juice. Season with freshly ground black pepper and process until well combined.

Put the fish in a flat, non-metallic dish and pour over the chermoula. Toss to coat well, cover and marinate in the refrigerator for 1 hour.

Bring a large saucepan of water to the boil and cook the potatoes for 10–12 minutes, or until cooked when tested with a skewer. Steam the zucchini and corn for 3 minutes, or until just cooked.

Meanwhile, remove the fish from the chermoula, reserving the liquid. Heat a chargrill plate or barbecue over a high heat and cook the fish for 2–3 minutes on each side, basting with the remaining chermoula. Serve immediately with the potatoes, zucchini and corn.

THIS LOW-FAT DISH IS A GOOD
CHOICE IF YOU'RE WATCHING
YOUR WEIGHT AS IT CONTAINS
HIGHLY FILLING FISH PROTEIN.

nutrition per serve: Energy 1656 kJ (396 Cal)
Fat 12.1 g
Saturated fat 1.6 g
Protein 34.4 g
Carbohydrate 31.9 g
Fibre 8.9 g
Cholesterol 78 mg
Sodium 151 mg

FISH TIKKA

WHY ORDER INDIAN TAKE-AWAY WHEN YOU CAN MAKE YOUR OWN? THIS TASTY
DISH IS EASY TO EAT AND SURE TO PLEASE THE WHOLE FAMILY.

MARINADE
250 g (9 oz/1 cup) low-fat plain yoghurt
2 spring onions (scallions), finely chopped
1 tbsp grated fresh ginger
2 garlic cloves, crushed
2 tbsp lemon juice
1 tsp ground coriander
1 tbsp garam masala
1 tsp paprika
1 tsp chilli powder
2 tbsp no-added-salt tomato paste
    (concentrated purée)

500 g (1 lb 2 oz) skinless firm white fish
    fillets (such as flake, sea bream, snapper,
    grouper or orange roughy)

2 onions, each cut into 8 chunks
2 small green or red capsicums (peppers),
    each cut into 8 chunks
boiled rice, to serve (optional)
lemon wedges, to serve

YOGHURT DRESSING
50 g (1¾ oz/about ⅓ cup) peeled, diced
    Lebanese (short) cucumber
1 tbsp chopped coriander (cilantro) leaves
250 g (9 oz/1 cup) low-fat plain yoghurt

PREP TIME: 25 MINUTES +
    1 HOUR MARINATING
COOKING TIME: 6 MINUTES
SERVES 4

Mix all the marinade ingredients together in a shallow non-metallic dish long enough and
deep enough to hold eight long metal skewers.

Cut the fish into 24 bite-sized chunks. On each skewer, thread 3 fish pieces, 2 onion
pieces and 2 capsicum pieces, alternating them as you go. Turn the skewers about in the
marinade so that all the fish and vegetables are well coated. Cover and marinate in the
refrigerator for at least 1 hour, or overnight if convenient.

Mix the yoghurt dressing ingredients together in a small bowl and set aside.

Heat the grill (broiler) to its highest setting. When the grill is very hot, lift the skewers out
of the marinade and grill for 5–6 minutes, or until the fish is firm and slightly charred.
Serve with the yoghurt dressing and lemon wedges.

nutrition per serve: Energy 1171 kJ (280 Cal); Fat 9; g; Saturated fat 4.3 g; Protein 33.2 g;
Carbohydrate 13.4 g; Fibre 3 g; Cholesterol 104 mg; Sodium 263 mg

BARBECUED PORK AND BROCCOLI

A CHINESE STREET-STALL CLASSIC CAN BE A HIT IN YOUR HOME TOO WITH THIS TASTY RECIPE.

2 tsp canola oil
1 large onion, thinly sliced
2 carrots, julienned
200 g (7 oz) broccoli, chopped
6 spring onions (scallions), diagonally sliced
1 tbsp finely chopped fresh ginger
3 garlic cloves, finely chopped
400 g (14 oz) Chinese barbecued pork, thinly sliced and trimmed of fat

1 tbsp reduced-sodium soy sauce
2 tbsp mirin
185 g (6½ oz/2 cups) bean sprouts
boiled basmati rice, to serve (optional)

PREP TIME: 25 MINUTES

TOTAL COOKING TIME: 10 MINUTES

SERVES 4

Heat a wok until very hot, add the oil and swirl it around to coat the side. Stir-fry the onion over medium heat for 3–4 minutes, or until slightly softened. Add the carrot, broccoli, spring onion, ginger and garlic and cook for 4–5 minutes, tossing the mixture constantly.

Increase the heat to high and add the barbecued pork. Toss constantly until the pork is well mixed with the vegetables and is heated through. Add the soy sauce and mirin, and toss until the ingredients are well coated. (The wok should be hot enough for the sauce to reduce into a glaze.) Add the bean sprouts and season with freshly ground black pepper. Serve immediately with the boiled rice.

HINT:
• Barbecued pork is available from Asian food stores.

nutrition per serve: Energy 1940 kJ (463 Cal); Fat 6.6; g; Saturated fat 1.5 g; Protein 28.6 g; Carbohydrate 65.4 g; Fibre 7.3 g; Cholesterol 54 mg; Sodium 546 mg

THIS LOW-CALORIE DISH IS
HIGH IN VITAMINS A AND C,
CALCIUM AND PROTEIN.

nutrition per serve: Energy 1452 g (347 Cal)

Fat 5.0 g

Saturated fat 1.2 g

Protein 38.0 g

Carbohydrate 35.2 g

Fibre 3.8 g

Cholesterol 97 g

Sodium 293 mg

LEMON GRASS CHICKEN AND RICE ROLLS

4 lemon grass stems, white part only,
  halved lengthways
3 boneless, skinless chicken breasts,
  halved lengthways
2 tsp sesame oil
2 red chillies, seeded and chopped
300 g (10½ oz) Chinese broccoli (gai larn),
  halved

300 g (10½ oz) plain rice noodle rolls
  (see Hint)
reduced-sodium soy sauce, to serve
lime wedges, to serve

PREP TIME: 15 MINUTES
COOKING TIME: 10 MINUTES
SERVES 4

Arrange the lemon grass in a steamer. Put the chicken on top, brush with the sesame oil and sprinkle with chilli. Cover with a lid. Sit the steamer over a wok or saucepan of boiling water and steam for 5 minutes, or until half cooked.

Put the Chinese broccoli and rice noodle rolls in another steamer of the same size and sit it on top of the steamer with the chicken. Cover with a lid and steam for a further 5 minutes, or until the chicken is cooked and the broccoli is tender. Cut the chicken into thick slices and serve with the broccoli, noodle rolls, small bowls of soy sauce and wedges of lime.

HINT:
• Rice noodle rolls are fresh blocks of thin rice noodles that have been rolled into a sausage shape. They are available from Asian food stores. If you cannot get them you can use fresh rice noodles, which are lower GI.

PEPPERED LAMB AND ASPARAGUS STIR-FRY WITH NOODLES

MUNG BEAN VERMICELLI IS LOW-GI AND TOGETHER WITH THE BEEF AND VEGETABLES, IS A GOOD CHOICE FOR PEOPLE WATCHING THEIR WEIGHT.

300 g (10½ oz) dried mung bean vermicelli
2 tsp green peppercorns, finely chopped
3 garlic cloves, finely chopped
2 tsp canola oil
400 g (14 oz) lean lamb fillets
canola oil spray
1 onion, cut into small wedges
4 tbsp dry sherry
1 green capsicum (pepper), cut into strips
200 g (7 oz) broccoli florets

16 small asparagus spears, trimmed and cut into bite-sized pieces
2 tbsp oyster sauce
garlic chives, cut into short lengths, to garnish

PREP TIME: 35 MINUTES + 20 MINUTES MARINATING + 10 MINUTES SOAKING
COOKING TIME: 30 MINUTES
SERVES 4

Put the noodles in a large bowl and cover with warm water. Soak for 10 minutes, or until they are translucent. Transfer to a saucepan of boiling water and cook for 15 minutes, or until tender. Rinse under cold water, then drain. Use scissors to cut into shorter lengths.

To make the marinade, put the green peppercorns, garlic and oil in a large non-metallic bowl. Add the lamb and toss well to coat. Cover with plastic wrap and marinate for 20 minutes.

Trim the lamb and cut into bite-sized pieces. Heat a wok over high heat until slightly smoking. Add the lamb in small batches and stir-fry briefly until browned and just cooked. Remove from the wok and keep warm. Reheat the wok between batches.

Reheat the wok, spray with oil and stir-fry the onion and 2 teaspoons of the sherry for 1 minute. Add the capsicum and a pinch of salt. Cover, steam for 2 minutes, add the broccoli, asparagus and the remaining sherry and stir-fry for 1 minute. Cover and steam for 3 minutes, or until the vegetables are just tender. Return the lamb to the pan, add the oyster sauce and stir to combine with the vegetables. Add the noodles and stir through until warmed. Serve garnished with the garlic chives.

HINT:
• People with diabetes or who are relatively inactive can serve themselves less vermicelli to for lower kilojoules.

nutrition per serve: Energy 2005 kJ (479 Cal); Fat 7 g; Saturated fat 1.9 g; Protein 25.4 g; Carbohydrate 70.2 g; Fibre 4.1 g; Cholesterol 65 mg; Sodium 582 mg

BEEF WITH OYSTER SAUCE

READY IN A FLASH—THIS DISH IS GREAT WHEN YOU WANT TO EAT
HEALTHY MEALS BUT HAVE LITTLE TIME FOR COOKING. THIS IS A
GOOD SOURCE OF PROTEIN.

1½ tsp cornflour (cornstarch)
125 ml (4 fl oz/½ cup) reduced-salt beef
   stock
1½ tbsp oyster sauce
1 tsp finely crushed garlic
1 tsp caster (superfine) sugar
2 tsp canola oil
350 g (12 oz) lean rump steak, finely sliced
250 g (9 oz) green beans, topped and
   tailed, cut into 5 cm (2 in) lengths

1 small red capsicum (pepper), sliced
60 g (2¼ oz/⅔ cup) bean sprouts
boiled basmati rice, to serve

PREP TIME: 15 MINUTES
TOTAL COOKING TIME: 10 MINUTES
SERVES 4

Dissolve the cornflour in a little of the stock. Mix with the remaining stock, oyster sauce,
garlic and sugar and set aside.

Heat the wok until very hot, add the oil and swirl it around to coat the side. Add the beef
in batches and stir-fry over high heat for 2 minutes, or until it browns.

Add the beans and capsicum and stir-fry another minute.

Add the cornflour mixture to the wok and cook until the sauce boils and thickens. Stir in
the bean sprouts and serve immediately with the rice.

nutrition per serve: Energy 1692 kJ (404 Cal); Fat 7.1 g; Saturated fat 2.1 g; Protein 26.7 g;
Carbohydrate 54.4 g; Fibre 3.1 g; Cholesterol 56 mg; Sodium 516 mg

JUNGLE PORK CURRY

CURRY PASTE
8–10 large dried red chillies
1 tbsp shrimp paste
1 tsp white pepper
1 lemon grass stem, white part only, sliced
5 red Asian shallots, sliced
5 garlic cloves, crushed
1 tbsp finely chopped galangal
2 tsp finely grated fresh ginger
2 small coriander (cilantro) roots, chopped

2 tsp canola oil
1 garlic clove, finely chopped, extra
500 g (1 lb 2 oz) lean pork fillet, thinly
   sliced
500 ml (17 fl oz/2 cups) reduced-salt
   chicken stock

½ tbsp reduced-sodium soy sauce
85 g (3 oz) Thai apple eggplants
   (aubergines), quartered, or Thai pea
   eggplants (aubergines)
100 g (3½ oz) snake (yard-long) beans,
   cut into 3 cm (1¼ in) lengths
60 g (2¼ oz/¼ cup) sliced bamboo shoots
4 makrut (kaffir lime) leaves, torn
1 small handful Thai basil leaves, plus extra
   to serve
1 long red chilli, seeded and julienned
boiled basmati rice, to serve

PREP TIME: 30 MINUTES + 10 MINUTES
SOAKING
TOTAL COOKING TIME: 20 MINUTES
SERVES 4

To make the curry paste, soak the dried chillies in boiling water for 10 minutes. Drain and chop. Wrap the shrimp paste in foil and toast in a hot wok for 1 minute on each side. Remove from the foil and put the shrimp paste in a food processor or blender with the chopped chilli and remaining paste ingredients. Process until smooth. Add a little water if necessary to form a smooth paste.

Heat a wok over medium heat, add the oil and swirl to coat. Add the garlic and 4 tablespoons of the curry paste and cook, stirring, for 1–2 minutes, or until fragrant. Add the pork and stir-fry for 2–3 minutes, or until browned. Pour in the stock and soy sauce, stir to combine, then bring to the boil. Add the eggplant, snake beans, bamboo shoots and lime leaves, reduce the heat and simmer for 5–8 minutes, or until the vegetables are tender but not soft. Remove from the heat and stir in the basil leaves. Garnish with the chilli strips and extra basil leaves and serve with the rice.

THIS AROMATIC THAI MEAL
PROVIDES PROTEIN, IRON AND
POTASSIUM. THE HOME-MADE
CURRY PASTE HAS LESS FAT
THAN COMMERCIAL VARIETIES.

nutrition per serve: Energy 1896 kJ (453 Cal)
Fat 6.5 g
Saturated fat 1.4 g
Protein 38.7 g
Carbohydrate 54.8 g
Fibre 5.5 g
Cholesterol 121 mg
Sodium 561 mg

BEEF IN BLACK BEAN SAUCE

THIS POPULAR CHINESE BEEF DISH SHOULD GIVE YOU AN ENERGY BOOST—
IT'S RICH IN IRON, ZINC AND CARBOHYDRATE.

2 garlic cloves, crushed

2 tsp grated fresh ginger

2 tbsp dry sherry

1 tbsp reduced-sodium soy sauce

750 g (1 lb 10 oz) lean beef rump steak

1 tsp cornflour (cornstarch)

2 tsp canola oil

2 onions, cut into wedges

1 large green capsicum (pepper), cut
   into strips

235 g (8½ oz) tin sliced bamboo shoots,
   drained and rinsed

2 tbsp tinned black beans, rinsed and
   chopped

boiled basmati rice, to serve

PREP TIME: 20 MINUTES + 1 HOUR
   MARINATING

COOKING TIME: 30 MINUTES

SERVES 4

To make the marinade, combine the garlic, ginger, sherry and soy sauce in a non-metallic bowl. Trim the meat, then slice across the grain into long, thin strips. Add to the marinade and toss to coat well. Cover with plastic wrap and refrigerate for at least 1 hour, turning occasionally. Drain the meat, reserving the marinade.

Meanwhile, to make the stir-fry sauce, mix the cornflour and remaining marinade with 2 tablespoons water until smooth.

Heat a wok until very hot, add half the oil and swirl to coat. Add the meat in small batches and stir-fry briefly until browned but not cooked through. Remove from the wok and drain on paper towels. Reheat the wok between batches.

Heat the remaining oil in the wok and swirl to coat. Add the onion and capsicum and stir-fry over high heat for 3 minutes, or until the onion is soft. Add the bamboo shoots and black beans, then cook for 1 minute.

Return the meat to the wok along with the stir-fry sauce and stir-fry over high heat until the meat is cooked through and the sauce has thickened. Serve immediately with the rice.

HINTS:
• Left-over black beans can be refrigerated for up to 2 weeks.
• For extra fibre and filling power, serve with brown rice instead of white rice.

nutrition per serve: Energy 2267 kJ (542 Cal); Fat 11.6 g; Saturated fat 4.1 g; Protein 60.4 g; Carbohydrate 54.5 g; Fibre 3.5 g; Cholesterol 120 mg; Sodium 308 mg

MIDDLE-EASTERN CHICKEN WITH BURGHUL

A NOURISHING MEAL THAT TASTES GREAT AND IS EASY TO MAKE, THIS DISH IS A GOOD WAY TO INCLUDE LOW-GI BURGHUL AND CHICKPEAS IN YOUR DIET.

350 g (12 oz/2 cups) burghul (bulgur)

2 skinless chicken breast fillets

2 tsp olive oil

1 red onion, thinly sliced

300 g (10½ oz) tin chickpeas, drained and rinsed

70 g (2½ oz/½ cup) unsalted pistachio kernels

1 tomato, chopped

juice of 1 orange

4 tbsp finely chopped flat-leaf (Italian) parsley

PREP TIME: 15 MINUTES + 15 MINUTES SOAKING

COOKING TIME: 20 MINUTES

SERVES 4

Put the burghul in a bowl, cover with water and leave to soak for 15 minutes, or until the burghul has softened. Drain and use clean hands to squeeze dry.

Meanwhile, trim the chicken and thinly slice. Heat a large frying pan over high heat, add half the oil and swirl to coat. Add the chicken in batches and stir-fry for 3–5 minutes, or until cooked. Remove from the pan and keep warm. Reheat the pan between batches.

Add the remaining oil to the pan and cook the onion, stirring, for 2 minutes, then add the chickpeas, pistachio kernels and tomato. Cook, stirring, for 3–5 minutes, or until the chickpeas are warmed through.

Pour in the orange juice, return the chicken and its juices to the pan and cook until half the juice has evaporated. Stir in the parsley. Season with freshly ground black pepper and serve with the burghul.

nutrition per serve: Energy 2457 kJ (589 Cal); Fat 13.7 g; Saturated fat 2.2 g; Protein 39.6 g; Carbohydrate 63.3 g; Fibre 20.7 g; Cholesterol 65 mg; Sodium 190 mg

THIS COLOURFUL DISH IS
GREAT IF YOU LOVE SEAFOOD.
PRAWNS PROVIDE PLENTY
OF PROTEIN WITH RELATIVELY
FEW KILOJOULES—BUT ENJOY
IN MODERATION AS THEY
CONTAIN CHOLESTEROL.

nutrition per serve: Energy 2121 kJ (507 Cal)
Fat 6.3 g
Saturated fat 0.9 g
Protein 38 g
Carbohydrate 69.3 g
Fibre 3.3 g
Cholesterol 226 mg
Sodium 547 mg

HONEY AND LIME PRAWN KEBABS WITH MANGO SALSA

MANGO SALSA
2 tomatoes
1 small just-ripe mango, diced
½ small red onion, diced
1 small red chilli, seeded and finely chopped
grated zest and juice of 1 lime
2 tbsp chopped coriander (cilantro) leaves

2 tbsp clear runny honey
1 small red chilli, seeded and finely chopped
1 tbsp olive oil

grated zest and juice of 2 limes
1 large garlic clove, crushed
2 cm (¾ in) piece fresh ginger, peeled and finely grated
1 tbsp chopped coriander (cilantro) leaves
32 tiger or king prawns (shrimp), peeled and deveined, tails intact
boiled rice, to serve

PREP TIME: 25 MINUTES + 30 MINUTES
SOAKING + 2 HOURS MARINATING
COOKING TIME: 5 MINUTES
SERVES 4

Before you start cooking, soak eight bamboo skewers in cold water for 30 minutes. While the skewers are soaking, make the salsa. Score a cross in the base of each tomato and put them in a heatproof bowl. Cover with boiling water, leave for 30 seconds, then plunge in cold water and peel the skin away from the cross. Remove the seeds, dice the flesh, saving any juices, and put the tomato with all its juices in a bowl. Mix in the mango, onion, chilli, lime zest, lime juice and coriander.

In a small bowl, whisk together the honey, chilli, oil, lime zest, lime juice, garlic, ginger and coriander. Put the prawns in a non-metallic dish, add the marinade and toss well. Cover and refrigerate for 2 or more hours, turning the prawns occasionally.

Heat the grill (broiler) to high. Thread 4 prawns onto each skewer and grill for 4 minutes, or until pink and cooked through, turning halfway through cooking and basting regularly with the left-over marinade. Serve at once with the salsa and the rice.

HINT:
• When threading the prawns on the skewers, don't squash them too closely together as they may not cook through properly.

FETTUCINE WITH SEARED TUNA AND ZUCCHINI

THIS LOW-FAT MEDITERRANEAN-STYLE DISH WITH A HINT OF ZESTY LEMON PROVIDES PLENTY OF PROTEIN, CARBOHYDRATE, NIACIN, POTASSIUM AND FOLATE, AND SOME IRON AND ZINC.

400 g (14 oz) fettucine pasta
500 g (1 lb 2 oz) tuna steaks
olive oil spray
1 large red onion, cut into thin wedges
2 zucchini (courgettes), sliced into 7 cm (2¾ in) long thin strips
1 garlic clove, chopped
6 small gherkins, rinsed and chopped

1 large handful flat-leaf (Italian) parsley, chopped
zest and juice of 1 large lemon
mixed-leaf salad, to serve (optional)

PREP TIME: 15 MINUTES
COOKING TIME: 20 MINUTES
SERVES 4

Cook the pasta in a large saucepan of boiling water for 10 minutes, or until *al dente*. Drain, reserving 250 ml (9 fl oz/1 cup) of the pasta water. Return the pasta to the saucepan.

Meanwhile, pat the fish dry with paper towels. Lightly spray a large, non-stick frying pan with the oil. Heat the oil, add the fish and cook for 2–3 minutes on each side, or until browned on the outside and still pink in the centre. Remove the fish from the pan. Set aside for a few minutes, then cut into 2 cm (¾ in) cubes.

Spray the frying pan with more oil and heat the pan. Add the onion, zucchini and garlic and cook for 2–3 minutes, or until softened. Stir in the gherkins, parsley, lemon zest and juice. Toss into the hot pasta together with the fish and enough of the reserved pasta water to moisten. Serve with a mixed-leaf salad.

nutrition per serve: Energy 2550 kJ (609 Cal); Fat 9.5 g; Saturated fat 3.3 g; Protein 45.8 g; Carbohydrate 80.2 g; Fibre 5.2 g; Cholesterol 63 mg; Sodium 271 mg

PASTA WITH MEATBALLS

THIS DELICIOUS DISH IS RICH IN SLOW-RELEASE CARBOHYDRATE AND
PROTEIN. LOW-GI, IT PROVIDES IRON AND ZINC, FOLATE AND POTASSIUM.

500 g (1 lb 2 oz) lean minced (ground) veal
1 onion, very finely chopped
4 garlic cloves, finely chopped
1 egg white, lightly beaten
80 g (2¾ oz/1 cup) fresh breadcrumbs
30 g (1 oz/½ cup) finely chopped parsley
7 g (¼ oz/¼ cup) finely chopped oregano
olive oil spray
1.5 kg (3 lb 5 oz) tomatoes, peeled, roughly chopped
2 onions, thinly sliced, extra

125 g (4½ oz/½ cup) no-added-salt tomato paste (concentrated purée)
½ tsp sugar
350 g (12 oz) penne
mixed-leaf salad, to serve (optional)

PREP TIME: 40 MINUTES
COOKING TIME: 1 HOUR 50 MINUTES
SERVES 6

Combine the minced veal, onion, half the garlic, egg white, breadcrumbs, two-thirds of the parsley and 1 tablespoon of the oregano. Season well. Mix with your hands until well combined. Shape into small balls.

Heat a frying pan and spray with oil. Cook the meatballs in three batches over high heat for 4–5 minutes, or until browned, turning constantly. Remove from the pan.

Lightly spray the base of a large, deep non-stick saucepan with oil. Add the sliced onion and remaining garlic. Cook over low heat for 2–3 minutes, stirring. Add 2 tablespoons water, cover and cook for 5 minutes. Stir in the tomatoes and tomato paste. Simmer, covered, for 10 minutes, then uncover and simmer gently for 40 minutes. Add the meatballs, and simmer, covered, for 15–20 minutes, or until just cooked. Add the sugar, remaining parsley and oregano, and season with freshly ground black pepper.

Cook the pasta in a large saucepan of boiling water for 10 minutes, or until *al dente*, then drain. Serve with the hot meatballs and the salad.

nutrition per serve: Energy 1901 kJ (454 Cal); Fat 8 g; Saturated fat 2.6 g; Protein 31.2 g; Carbohydrate 59.2 g; Fibre 7 g; Cholesterol 68 mg; Sodium 213 mg

PENNE WITH BACON, RICOTTA AND BASIL SAUCE

2 tsp olive oil

4 low-fat back bacon slices (we used 97% fat-free), chopped

2–3 garlic cloves, crushed

1 onion, finely chopped

2 spring onions (scallions), finely chopped

250 g (9 oz/1 cup) low-fat ricotta cheese

3 handfuls basil, finely chopped, plus extra whole leaves, to garnish

325 g (11½ oz) penne

12 cherry tomatoes, halved

PREP TIME: 20 MINUTES

COOKING TIME: 15 MINUTES

SERVES 4

Heat the oil in a frying pan, add the bacon, garlic, onion and spring onion and stir over medium heat for 5 minutes, or until cooked. Remove from the heat, stir in the ricotta and chopped basil and beat until smooth.

Cook the pasta in a large saucepan of boiling water for 10 minutes, or until *al dente*. Just prior to draining the pasta, add about 250 ml (9 fl oz/1 cup) of the pasta cooking water to the ricotta mixture to thin the sauce. Add more water if you prefer an even thinner sauce. Season with freshly ground black pepper.

Drain the pasta and stir the ricotta sauce and tomato halves through the pasta. Garnish with extra basil and serve.

DELICIOUS FRESHLY PREPARED
BUT ALSO WHEN SERVED AS
LEFTOVERS, THIS ITALIAN
MEAL IS RICH IN FLAVOUR
AND NUTRIENTS.

nutrition per serve: Energy 1700 kJ (406 Cal)
Fat 7.2 g
Saturated fat 2.1 g
Protein 21.3 g
Carbohydrate 61.7 g
Fibre 4.7 g
Cholesterol 8 mg
Sodium 516 mg

CHICKEN AND VEGETABLE LASAGNE

A REAL CROWD PLEASER, THIS VERSION OF LASAGNE IS MADE WITH CHICKEN AND LOTS OF VEGETABLES. IT'S LOW-GI AND CONTAINS MUCH LESS FAT THAN TRADITIONAL LASAGNE.

500 g (1 lb 2 oz) chicken breast fillets
olive oil spray
2 garlic cloves, crushed
1 onion, chopped
2 zucchini (courgettes), chopped
2 celery stalks, chopped
2 carrots, chopped
300 g (10½ oz) pumpkin (winter squash), diced
2 x 400 g (14 oz) tins reduced-salt diced tomatoes
2 sprigs thyme
2 bay leaves
2 tbsp no-added-salt tomato paste (concentrated purée)

125 ml (4 fl oz/½ cup) dry white wine
2 tbsp chopped basil
500 g (1 lb 2 oz) English spinach
500 g (1 lb 2 oz) low-fat cottage cheese
450 g (1 lb) low-fat ricotta cheese
60 ml (2 fl oz/¼ cup) skim milk
½ tsp ground nutmeg
35 g (1¼ oz/⅓ cup) grated parmesan cheese
300 g (10½ oz) lasagne sheets

PREP TIME: 45 MINUTES

TOTAL COOKING TIME: 1 HOUR 20 MINUTES

SERVES 8

Preheat the oven to 180°C (350°F/Gas 4). Trim any excess fat from the chicken breasts, then finely mince in a food processor. Heat a large, deep, non-stick frying pan, spray lightly with oil and cook the chicken mince in batches until browned. Set aside. Add the garlic and onion to the pan and cook until softened. Return the chicken to the pan and add the zucchini, celery, carrot, pumpkin, tomato, thyme, bay leaves, tomato paste and wine. Simmer, covered, for 20 minutes. Remove the bay leaves and thyme, stir in the fresh basil and set aside.

Shred the spinach and set aside. Mix the cottage cheese, ricotta, skim milk, nutmeg and half the parmesan. Spoon a little of the tomato mixture over the base of a casserole dish and top with a single layer of pasta, top with half the remaining tomato mixture, then the spinach and spoon over half the cottage cheese mixture. Continue with another layer of pasta. Spread the remaining tomato mixture then the cottage cheese on top and sprinkle with parmesan. Bake for 40–50 minutes, or until golden. The top may puff up slightly but will settle on standing.

nutrition per serve: Energy 1719 kJ (411 Cal); Fat 7.5 g; Saturated fat 3.2 g; Protein 40.4 g; Carbohydrate 39.7 g; Fibre 6.3 g; Cholesterol 53 mg; Sodium 299 mg

ITALIAN FISH ROLLS WITH SWEET POTATO

THIS FLAVOURSOME MEAL IS A DELICIOUS WAY TO EAT FISH AND IS A GOOD SOURCE OF PROTEIN, IODINE, SELENIUM, BETA-CAROTENE AND B-GROUP VITAMINS. IT IS LOW-GI AND VERY LOW IN FAT.

1 large tomato

1 tbsp capers, drained and chopped

45 g (1½ oz/¼ cup) stuffed green olives in brine, drained and chopped

3 tbsp finely chopped lemon thyme

30 g (1 oz/¼ cup) finely grated romano cheese

2 tsp finely grated lemon zest

¼ tsp freshly ground black pepper

8 thin white skinless fish fillets (about 850 g/1 lb 14 oz) (see Hint)

250 ml (9 fl oz/1 cup) dry white wine

2 tbsp lemon juice

3 tbsp lemon thyme, extra

2 bay leaves

800 g (1 lb 12 oz) sweet potato, peeled and cut into 5 cm (2 in) pieces

PREP TIME: 30 MINUTES

COOKING TIME: 30 MINUTES

SERVES 4–6

Preheat the oven to 160°C (315°F/Gas 2–3). Peel and chop the tomato and score a cross in the base. Cover with boiling water for 30 seconds, then plunge into cold water. Drain and peel away the skin from the cross. Cut in half and scoop out the seeds. Roughly chop the flesh and mix with the capers, olives, lemon thyme, cheese, lemon zest and freshly ground pepper in a small bowl.

Put the fillets, skinned side up, on a flat surface. Spread the tomato mixture evenly onto each fillet, then roll up tightly and secure with a toothpick or skewer. Place in a single layer in a shallow casserole dish.

Pour the combined wine, juice, lemon thyme and bay leaves over the fish, cover with foil and bake for 20 minutes, or until the fish is cooked and flakes easily when tested with a fork.

Meanwhile, cook the sweet potato in a large saucepan of boiling water for 10 minutes or until cooked. Drain and roughly mash. Season with freshly ground black pepper. Serve with the fish rolls.

HINT:
• Use john dory, bream, perch or snapper or ask your fishmonger for a suggestion.

nutrition per serve (6): Energy 1175 kJ (281 Cal); Fat 5.1 g; Saturated fat 1.9 g; Protein 31.1 g; Carbohydrate 18.3 g; Fibre 3.9 g; Cholesterol 78 mg; Sodium 366 mg

THIS TASTY DISH IS A GREAT
WAY TO INCLUDE THE
NUTRITIONAL BENEFITS OF
SALMON IN YOUR DIET. IT
CONTAINS OMEGA-3 FATTY
ACIDS, PROTEIN, POTASSIUM
AND PHOSPHORUS.

nutrition per serve: Energy 1274 kJ (304 Cal)
Fat 16.2 g
Saturated fat 3 g
Protein 26.9 g
Carbohydrate 10.4 g
Fibre 4.4 g
Cholesterol 65 mg
Sodium 171 mg

GRILLED SALMON WITH FENNEL AND ORANGE SALAD

FENNEL AND ORANGE SALAD
1 fennel bulb, with fronds
2 oranges, peeled and segmented
12 pitted black olives
1 tbsp snipped chives
1½ tbsp virgin olive oil
1 tbsp lemon juice
½ tsp dijon mustard
¼ tsp caster (superfine) sugar

500 g (1 lb 2 oz) piece salmon fillet
olive oil spray
200 g (7 oz) baby English spinach leaves

PREP TIME: 20 MINUTES

COOKING TIME: 2 MINUTES

SERVES 4

To prepare the salad, trim the fronds from the fennel bulb and finely chop up enough fronds to fill a tablespoon. Remove the stalks from the fennel and cut a 5 mm (¼ in) thick slice off the base of the bulb. Cut the bulb in half, then finely slice and toss in a large bowl with the chopped fronds, orange segments, olives and chives. In a separate bowl, whisk the oil with the lemon juice, mustard and sugar. Season to taste with freshly ground black pepper, pour over the fennel mixture and toss gently to coat.

Heat the grill (broiler) to medium. Remove the bones and skin from the salmon and cut the flesh into 1 cm (½ in) thick slices. Lightly spray a grill tray with oil, put on the salmon slices, spray with more oil and season with freshly ground black pepper. Grill for 1–2 minutes, or until just cooked through.

Divide the spinach leaves among four large serving plates, top with the fennel and orange salad and arrange the salmon over the spinach. Serve warm.

HINT:
• Fennel bulbs are easily sliced using the slicing disc of a food processor.

115

LAMB CUTLETS WITH CANNELLINI BEAN PUREE

LEGUMES LIKE CANNELLINI BEANS ARE A GREAT FOOD TO INCLUDE IN A LOWER FAT DIET TO CONTROL YOUR BLOOD CHOLESTEROL BECAUSE THEY ARE LOW-GI, LOW IN FAT AND CHOLESTEROL FREE.

8 lean lamb cutlets

4 garlic cloves

1 tbsp chopped rosemary

2 tsp olive oil

2 x 400 g (14 oz) tins cannellini beans, drained

1 tsp ground cumin

125 ml (4 fl oz/½ cup) lemon juice

olive oil spray

2 tbsp balsamic vinegar

PREP TIME: 30 MINUTES + 1 HOUR REFRIGERATION

TOTAL COOKING TIME: 10 MINUTES

SERVES 4

Trim the cutlets of excess fat from the outside edge and scrape the fat away from the bones. Put in a single layer in a shallow dish. Thinly slice 2 garlic cloves and mix with the rosemary, oil and some freshly ground black pepper. Pour over the meat, cover and refrigerate for 1 hour.

Rinse the beans and purée with the remaining garlic, the cumin and half the lemon juice in a food processor or blender. Transfer to a pan, then set aside.

Lightly spray a non-stick frying pan with oil and cook the cutlets over medium heat for 1–2 minutes on each side. Add the vinegar and cook for 1 minute, turning to coat. Remove the cutlets and cover to keep warm. Add the remaining lemon juice to the pan and simmer for 2–3 minutes, or until the sauce thickens slightly. Warm the purée over medium heat and serve with the cutlets.

nutrition per serve: Energy 1307 kJ (312 Cal); Fat 11.6 g; Saturated fat 4.3 g; Protein 29.2 g; Carbohydrate 18.4 g; Fibre 9.3 g; Cholesterol 60 mg; Sodium 71 mg

STEAK SANDWICH WITH ONION RELISH

THIS IS ONE HEARTY (AND TASTY) SANDWICH THAT'S PACKED WITH LOTS OF NUTRIENTS, SUCH AS PROTEIN, NIACIN, PHOSPHORUS AND EASILY ABSORBED ZINC AND IRON.

RED ONION RELISH
1 tsp olive oil
2 red onions, thinly sliced
2 tbsp soft brown sugar
2 tbsp balsamic vinegar
1 tbsp chopped thyme

250 g (9 oz) mixed mushrooms (flat, button, shiitake), sliced
olive oil spray

4 lean minute beef steaks, trimmed
3 large handfuls baby English spinach leaves
ciabatta or sourdough bread
mixed-leaf salad, to serve (optional)

PREP TIME: 20 MINUTES
COOKING TIME: 25 MINUTES
SERVES 4

To make the red onion relish, heat the oil in a saucepan. Add the onion and cook over a low heat for 10 minutes, or until softened, taking care not to burn. Add the sugar and balsamic vinegar. Cook and stir often over a low heat for 10–12 minutes, or until softened and slightly syrupy. Stir in the thyme.

Meanwhile, put the mushrooms and 125 ml (4 fl oz/½ cup) water in a heavy-based frying pan. Bring to the boil, stirring to coat the mushrooms in the water. Simmer, covered, for 5 minutes, or until softened, making sure the mushrooms don't dry out. Stir once or twice. Remove the lid and increase the heat to allow the juice to evaporate. Season with freshly ground black pepper.

Lightly spray a chargrill pan or frying pan with the oil. Add the meat and cook for 1 minute on each side, or until cooked to your liking.

Very briefly microwave or steam the spinach until just wilted. Drain away any juices.

Slice the bread on the diagonal into 8 thick slices and toast. To serve, arrange 2 slices of bread on each plate. Top with the spinach, then the steak and mushrooms and finish with a dollop of the relish. Serve with a mixed-leaf salad to boost your intake of antioxidants.

nutrition per serve: Energy 1819 kJ (435 Cal); Fat 9.8 g; Saturated fat 3.2 g; Protein 41.3 g; Carbohydrate 41.7 g; Fibre 6.2 g; Cholesterol 85 mg; Sodium 477 mg

SHISH KEBABS WITH RISONI SALAD

200 g (7 oz/1 cup) risoni
2 tsp extra virgin olive oil
2 tsp balsamic vinegar
½ tsp grated lemon zest
2 tsp lemon juice
40 g (1¾ oz) baby rocket (arugula) leaves
1½ tbsp shredded basil
½ small red onion, finely sliced

SHISH KEBABS
250 g (9 oz) lean minced (ground) lamb
250 g (9 oz) minced (ground) veal

1 onion, finely chopped
2 garlic cloves, crushed
1 tsp ground allspice
1 tsp ground cinnamon
olive oil spray

PREP TIME: 25 MINUTES + 30 MINUTES
   REFRIGERATION TIME
COOKING TIME: 20 MINUTES
SERVES 4

First, make the risoni salad. Bring a saucepan of water to the boil, add the risoni and cook for about 12 minutes, or until tender. Drain, rinse under cold water, then drain again. Put the risoni in a large bowl with the oil, vinegar, lemon zest, lemon juice, rocket, basil and onion. Mix well, season to taste with freshly ground black pepper and refrigerate until ready to serve.

To make the shish kebabs, put the lamb, veal, onion, garlic, allspice and cinnamon in a food processor or blender with a little pepper. Process until fine, but not mushy. Divide the mixture into eight equal portions, then roll into long sausage-shaped shish kebabs. Insert a long metal skewer through the middle of each shish kebab, pressing the mixture firmly onto the skewers. Refrigerate for 30 minutes to firm.

Preheat a barbecue grill plate, flat plate or chargrill pan to medium. Spray the hotplate with oil and grill the kebabs for about 8–10 minutes, or until cooked through, turning often. Serve warm with the risoni salad.

THESE MIDDLE-EASTERN
KEBABS ARE SURE TO BE A
FAVOURITE WITH THE WHOLE
FAMILY. THEY ARE HIGH IN
PROTEIN, LOW-GI AND A GOOD
SOURCE OF IRON AND ZINC.

nutrition per serve: Energy 1675 kJ (400 Cal)
Fat 12.5 g
Saturated fat 4.2 g
Protein 32.9 g
Carbohydrate 36.9 g
Fibre 3 g
Cholesterol 94 mg
Sodium 111 mg

119

VEAL GOULASH

THIS TRADITIONAL HEARTY HUNGARIAN STEW IS A REAL CROWD PLEASER.
SLOW-COOKED WITH THE COMPLEX TASTE AND AROMA OF PAPRIKA, IT IS A
GREAT DISH TO COOK AND ENJOY ON A LAZY WEEKEND.

500 g (1 lb 2 oz) veal, cut into 2.5 cm
  (1 in) pieces
2 tbsp plain (all-purpose) flour
1 tbsp olive oil

olive oil spray
2 onions thinly sliced
2 garlic cloves, chopped
1 tbsp sweet Hungarian paprika
1 tsp ground cumin
440 g (15½ oz) tin reduced-salt diced
  tomatoes
2 carrots, sliced

½ red capsicum (pepper), chopped
½ green capsicum (pepper), chopped
250 ml (9 fl oz/1 cup) reduced-salt beef
  stock
125 ml (4 fl oz/½ cup) red wine
125 g (4 fl oz/½ cup) extra-light sour
  cream
chopped parsley, to garnish

PREP TIME: 25 MINUTES

TOTAL COOKING: TIME 2 HOURS

SERVES 4

Put the veal and flour in a plastic bag and shake to coat the veal. Shake off any excess flour. Heat the oil in a large deep heavy-based pan over medium heat. Brown the meat well in batches, then remove the meat and set aside.

Reheat the pan and spray with olive oil. Cook the onion, garlic, paprika and cumin for 5 minutes, stirring frequently. Return the meat and any juices to the pan with the tomato, carrot and capsicum. Cook and cover for 10 minutes.

Add the stock and wine and season with freshly ground black pepper. Stir well, then cover and simmer over very low heat for 1½ hours. Stir in half the sour cream, season with more pepper if needed and serve garnished with parsley and the remaining sour cream.

HINT:
• This dish is delicious served with boiled new potatoes or noodles.

nutrition per serve: Energy 1421 kJ (340 Cal); Fat 12.5 g; Saturated fat 4.2 g; Protein 33.3 g; Carbohydrate 16.1 g; Fibre 4.3 g; Cholesterol 103 mg; Sodium 424 mg

GIANT SALMON BALLS

YOU'LL BE BOWLED OVER BY THESE TASTY SALMON BALLS BECAUSE THEY
ARE OVEN-BAKED AND NOT DEEP-FRIED. TEAM THEM WITH A SALAD AND MAKE
A MEAL OF THEM.

3 potatoes, cut into 5 cm (2 in) cubes
100 g (3½ oz/½ cup) long-grain rice
50 g (1¾ oz/½ cup) rolled (porridge) oats
415 g (14¾ oz) tin red salmon in spring
    water, drained and flaked
1 egg, lightly beaten
3 spring onions (scallions), chopped
2 tbsp lemon juice
2 tbsp sweet chilli sauce
80 g (2¾ oz/1 cup) fresh breadcrumbs

2 eggs, lightly beaten, extra
200 g (7 oz/2 cups) dry breadcrumbs
olive oil spray
lemon wedges, to serve
mixed-leaf salad, to serve

PREP TIME: 35 MINUTES + 30 MINUTES
    REFRIGERATION
COOKING TIME: 40 MINUTES
MAKES 8 BALLS

Boil, steam or microwave the potatoes until tender. Drain, mash and set aside to cool.
Cook the rice in a saucepan of boiling water for 10 minutes, or until tender. Drain and cool.

Put the potato, rice, oats, salmon, egg, spring onions, lemon juice, chilli sauce and fresh
breadcrumbs in a bowl, and mix together well. Season with freshly ground black pepper.

Divide the mixture into 8 portions and shape into balls. Dip in the egg, then in the dry
breadcrumbs. Place on a baking tray lined with baking paper, cover and refrigerate for
30 minutes.

Preheat the oven to 200°C (400°F/Gas 6). Spray the salmon balls lightly with the oil and
bake for 30 minutes, or until crisp, golden and heated through. Serve with lemon wedges
and a large mixed-leaf salad.

nutrition per serve: Energy 1437 kJ (343 Cal); Fat 9 g; Saturated fat 2.3 g; Protein 18 g;
Carbohydrate 45.3 g; Fibre 3.2 g; Cholesterol 96 mg; Sodium 348 mg

THESE CHICKEN SCHNITZELS HAVE A TOUCH OF THE EXOTIC ABOUT THEM, COATED IN HERBS AND SPICES RATHER THAN BREADCRUMBS.

nutrition per serve: Energy 2160 kJ (516 Cal)
Fat 8.9 g
Saturated fat 2.1 g
Protein 56.9 g
Carbohydrate 48.8 g
Fibre 3.7 g
Cholesterol 133 mg
Sodium 283 mg

SPICY CHICKEN SCHNITZELS

4 x 200 g (7 oz) chicken breast fillets
½ tbsp ground coriander
½ tbsp ground cumin
¼ tsp chilli powder, or to taste
1 garlic clove, crushed
1 tbsp lemon juice
1 tbsp olive oil
250 g (9 oz/1 cup) low-fat plain yoghurt
½ tsp harissa paste, or to taste
½ tsp caster (superfine) sugar
2 tbsp finely chopped mint leaves, plus
   extra sprigs, to serve

COUSCOUS SALAD
185 g (6½ oz/1 cup) couscous
300 g (10½ oz) tin chickpeas, rinsed and
   drained
75 g (2½ oz) cherry tomatoes, halved
½ small red onion, thinly sliced

PREP TIME: 25 MINUTES + 15 MINUTES
   STANDING
COOKING TIME: 10 MINUTES
SERVES 4

Put the chicken breasts between two sheets of plastic wrap and flatten them with a mallet or rolling pin until 1½ cm (⅝ in) thick.

In a small bowl, mix the ground coriander, cumin, chilli powder, garlic, lemon juice and oil together to form a paste. Thoroughly rub the paste all over the chicken fillets, then cover and leave to stand for 10 minutes.

To make the couscous salad, pour 250 ml (9 fl oz/1 cup) boiling water over the in couscous in a bowl. Cover with plastic wrap and leave for 5 minutes then fluff up with a fork. Stir through chick peas, tomatoes and onion slices.

Heat the grill (broiler) to high. Put the chicken on a lightly oiled grill tray and grill for 6–8 minutes, or until cooked through, turning once.

Meanwhile, blend 1 tablespoon of the yoghurt in a bowl with the harissa and sugar. Stir in the remaining yoghurt and mint, season to taste with freshly ground black pepper.

Garnish the chicken with the extra mint sprigs and serve with the yoghurt mix and couscous.

HINT:
• These schnitzels are also delicious served cold or eaten in a wholegrain bread roll
  as a burger.

STUFFED BEEF FILLET

THIS NOURISHING DISH SHOWS HOW EASY IT IS TO EAT A VARIETY OF VEGETABLES IN ONE MEAL. IT'S A GOOD SOURCE OF PROTEIN, B GROUP VITAMINS, IRON AND ZINC.

1 tsp olive oil

2 French shallots, finely chopped

60 g (2¼ oz) mushrooms, finely chopped

20 g (¾ oz/½ cup) fresh wholemeal (whole-wheat) breadcrumbs

1 tbsp thyme

1 tbsp wholegrain mustard

olive oil spray

600 g (1 lb 5 oz) lean beef fillet

800 g (1 lb 12 oz) new potatoes, cut into bite-sized chunks

4 corn cobs, each cut in 4 pieces

SAUCE

1 tsp orange zest

185 ml (6 fl oz/¾ cup) orange juice

1 tbsp orange marmalade

1 tbsp wholegrain mustard

PREP TIME: 30 MINUTES

COOKING TIME: 55 MINUTES

SERVES 4

Preheat the oven to 190°C (375°F/Gas 5). Heat the oil in a non-stick frying pan. Cook the shallots and mushrooms for 2 minutes, or until slightly softened. Put in a small bowl with the breadcrumbs and thyme leaves. Mix in the mustard and 2 teaspoons water to just moisten.

Cut along one side of the fillet to open out or create a butterfly. Spread the mushroom mixture over the surface. Enclose the filling and tie, at intervals, with string. Pat the meat dry with paper towels. Spray a heavy-based frying pan with oil. Heat and add the beef and cook on a high heat until browned all over. Put in a roasting tin. Roast for 25 minutes, or until cooked to your liking. Remove the meat from the oven, cover with foil and rest. Remove the string.

Meanwhile, line a baking tray with baking paper. Put the potatoes in a large saucepan of boiling water. Cook for 5 minutes, or until partially cooked. Drain well. Put the potatoes on the prepared tray. Season with freshly ground black pepper and spray with oil. Bake for 15–20 minutes, or until crisp and cooked through. Cook the corn cobs in a saucepan of boiling water for 8 minutes, or until tender. Drain.

Add the sauce ingredients to the roasting tin. Stir to dissolve the marmalade and allow it to reduce a little. To serve, thickly slice the meat. Arrange the meat on plates, drizzle over a little of the sauce and serve with the potatoes and corn.

nutrition per serve: Energy 2056 kJ (491 Cal); Fat 10.9 g; Saturated fat 3.6 g; Protein 40.3 g; Carbohydrate 52.8 g; Fibre 7.8 g; Cholesterol 100 mg; Sodium 199 mg

REDUCED-FAT MOUSSAKA

THIS REDUCED-FAT VERSION OF A GREEK FAVOURITE MAKES A NOURISHING,
LOW-GI MEAL.

1 kg (2 lb 4 oz) eggplant (aubergine)
olive oil spray
2 onions, finely chopped
3 large garlic cloves, crushed
½ tsp ground allspice
1 tsp ground cinnamon
500 g (1 lb 2 oz) lean minced (ground) lamb
2 tbsp no-added-salt tomato paste
    (concentrated purée)
125 ml (4 fl oz/½ cup) red wine
2 x 400 g (14 oz) tins reduced-salt
    tomatoes

3 tbsp chopped parsley
90 g (3¼ oz) low-fat cheddar cheese
20 g (¾ oz) olive or canola oil margarine
40 g (1½ oz/⅓ cup) plain flour
375 ml (13 fl oz/1½ cups) skim milk
150 g (5½ oz/⅔ cup) low-fat ricotta
pinch ground nutmeg

PREP TIME: 30 MINUTES
COOKING TIME: 1½ HOURS
SERVES 6

Preheat the oven to 180°C (350°F/Gas 4). Cut the eggplant into 5 mm (¼ in) thick slices. Spray the eggplant with the oil and grill (broil) under a preheated grill (broiler) for 4 minutes on each side, or until golden.

Heat a large, non-stick saucepan and lightly spray with oil. Cook the onions for 3–4 minutes, or until softened. Add the garlic, allspice and cinnamon and cook for 1 minute. Add the lamb and cook for 3–4 minutes, or until cooked. Add the tomato paste, wine and tomatoes. Bring to the boil, then reduce the heat and simmer for 30–35 minutes, stirring occasionally, or until most of the liquid has evaporated. Stir in the parsley and season with freshly ground black pepper.

To make the white sauce, grate the cheese. Melt the margarine in a saucepan over a medium heat. Stir in the flour and cook for 1 minute. Remove from the heat and gradually stir in the milk. Return to the heat and stir constantly until the sauce boils and thickens. Reduce the heat and simmer for 2 minutes. Stir through the ricotta and nutmeg until smooth and season with pepper.

Spoon half the meat sauce over the base of a 3 litre (105 fl oz/12 cup) 25 x 30 cm (10 x 12 in) ovenproof dish. Cover with half of the eggplant. Spoon over the remaining meat sauce and cover with the remaining eggplant. Spread over the sauce and sprinkle with the cheese. Bake for 30 minutes, or until golden. Stand for 5 minutes before serving.

nutrition per serve: Energy 1451 kJ (347 Cal); Fat 12.2 g; Saturated fat 4.4 g; Protein 31.4 g; Carbohydrate 20.8 g; Fibre 7.1 g; Cholesterol 65 mg; Sodium 282 mg

POACHED SALMON KEDGEREE

2 eggs
750 ml (26 fl oz/3 cups) reduced-salt fish or
 chicken stock
125 ml (4 fl oz/½ cup) dry white wine
½ lemon, sliced
2 x 200 g (7 oz) salmon fillets
1 tsp canola oil margarine
1 large red onion, chopped
2 tbsp mild curry powder
2 tsp ground turmeric
300 g (10½ oz/1½ cups) basmati rice
60 g (2¼ oz/½ cup) sultanas
 (golden raisins)

1 large handful flat-leaf (Italian) parsley,
 finely chopped
1 lemon, cut into 4 wedges, to serve
 (optional)
ready-made fruit chutney, to serve
 (optional)
mixed-leaf salad, to serve (optional)

PREP TIME: 20 MINUTES
COOKING TIME: 40 MINUTES
SERVES 4

Put the eggs in a saucepan, cover with water and bring to the boil. Boil for 5 minutes, drain and cool quickly in cold water. Peel and chop roughly.

Heat a heavy-based frying pan that is 8 cm (3 in) deep and 24 cm (9½ in) in diameter across the base. Add the stock, wine and lemon slices and heat, then add the fish. Lower the heat and simmer for 8 minutes, or until just cooked through. Place the fish on a plate, remove the skin and roughly flake with a fork. Strain the stock into a jug to measure 750 ml (26 fl oz/3 cups). Set aside. Wipe out the pan.

Heat the butter in the frying pan, add the onion and cook for 2 minutes, or until softened. Add the curry powder, the turmeric and rice. Stir to combine and cook for 1 minute.

Stir in the reserved stock. Bring to the boil, lower the heat, cover and simmer for 20 minutes, or until the rice is cooked and the liquid has been absorbed.

Gently stir the chopped egg, fish, sultanas and half of the parsley through the rice. Top with the remaining parsley and lemon wedges on the side, if using. Serve with a little fruit chutney and a mixed-leaf salad.

A SPICED DISH COMBINING
GOOD-QUALITY PROTEIN FROM
EGGS AND SALMON WITH LOW-GI
CARBOHYDRATE FROM BASMATI RICE.
THIS MEAL ALSO PROVIDES SOME
IRON, ESSENTIAL OMEGA-3 FATTY
ACIDS, NIACIN AND POTASSIUM.

nutrition per serve: Energy 2380 kJ (569 Cal)
Fat 11.3 g
Saturated fat 2.7 g
Protein 32.2 g
Carbohydrate 77.2 g
Fibre 3.4 g
Cholesterol 149 mg
Sodium 572 mg

SHEPHERD'S PIE

A REDUCED-FAT VERSION OF AN OLD FAVOURITE, THIS HEARTY PIE IS JUST AS DELICIOUS AS THE REGULAR VERSION.

1 kg (2 lb 4 oz) potatoes
6 large garlic cloves, peeled
4 tbsp skim milk
olive oil spray
1 large onion, finely chopped
3 large garlic cloves, crushed
2 celery sticks, finely chopped
2 carrots, diced
750 g (1 lb 10 oz) lean minced (ground) lamb
1½ tbsp plain (all-purpose) flour
2 tbsp no-added-salt tomato paste (concentrated purée)

2 tsp chopped thyme
2 tsp chopped rosemary
2 bay leaves
315 ml (10¾ fl oz/1¼ cups) reduced-salt beef stock
1 tbsp worcestershire sauce
pinch ground nutmeg
mixed-leaf salad, to serve (optional)

PREP TIME: 20 MINUTES
COOKING TIME: 45 MINUTES
SERVES 6

Preheat the oven to 180°C (350°F/Gas 4). Cut the potatoes into chunks and cook in a large saucepan of boiling water with the whole garlic cloves for 10–15 minutes, or until tender. Drain well and return to the saucepan. Mash the potato and garlic with a potato masher until smooth. Stir through the milk and season with freshly ground black pepper.

Heat a frying pan over medium heat, then spray with oil. Add the onion, crushed garlic, celery and carrot and cook for 5 minutes, or until the vegetables begin to soften (add water if needed). Remove from the pan.

Add the lamb and cook over a high heat until well browned, breaking up any lumps with the back of a spoon. Add the flour and cook for 1–2 minutes. Return the vegetables to the pan with the tomato paste, herbs, bay leaf, stock, sauce and nutmeg and bring to the boil. Reduce the heat and simmer for 5 minutes, or until thickened.

Pour the lamb mixture into a 2 litre (70 fl oz/4 cup) ovenproof dish. Spoon the potato over the top, smoothing the surface, then fluff with a fork. Bake for 25–30 minutes, or until lightly golden and crusty. Serve with a mixed-leaf salad.

nutrition per serve: Energy 1495 kJ (357 Cal); Fat 9.8 g; Saturated fat 4.1 g; Protein 32.9 g; Carbohydrate 30.7 g; Fibre 5.6 g; Cholesterol 87 mg; Sodium 383 mg

MEATLOAF

PREPARING A FAMILY DINNER DOESN'T HAVE TO BE HARD WORK. MEATLOAF IS A GREAT WAY TO GET CHILDREN TO EAT VEGETABLES—SIMPLY GRATE THEM AND ADD THEM TO THE MIXTURE WHERE THEY WILL HARDLY BE NOTICED.

60 g (2¼ oz) sweet potato
1 carrot
canola or olive oil spray
2 onions, finely chopped
2 garlic cloves, crushed
125 g (4½ oz/1½ cups) fresh wholegrain
   breadcrumbs
2 tbsp chopped parsley
500 g (1 lb 2 oz) lean minced (ground) beef
2 tbsp worcestershire sauce
1 tsp dried basil
1 tbsp no-added-salt tomato paste
   (concentrated purée)

300 g (10½ oz) tin chickpeas, drained
   and rinsed
1 egg, lightly beaten
90 g (3¼ oz/1 cup) button mushrooms,
   thinly sliced
400 g (14 oz) tin reduced-salt tomatoes
1 tbsp dry white wine
1 tsp soft brown sugar
mixed leaf salad, to serve

PREP TIME: 20 MINUTES
COOKING TIME: 1 HOUR 20 MINUTES
SERVES 6

Preheat the oven to 200°C (400°F/Gas 6). Coarsely grate the sweet potato and carrot.

Heat a non-stick frying pan over medium heat, then spray with the oil. Add the onion and cook, stirring, for 2 minutes. Add 1 tablespoon water to prevent sticking, then add the garlic and stir for 3 minutes, or until the onion is golden brown. Set aside to cool completely.

Use your hands to thoroughly mix together the breadcrumbs, parsley, beef, Worcestershire sauce, basil, tomato paste, grated sweet potato and carrot and the cooled onion mixture. Mix in the chickpeas, egg and mushrooms. Season with freshly ground black pepper. Transfer to a 10 x 18 cm (4 x 7 in) non-stick loaf tin (or loaf tin lined with baking paper), pressing gently into the tin and smoothing the top.

To make the tomato sauce, push the undrained tomatoes through a sieve, then discard the contents of the sieve. Add the wine and sugar to the tomato mixture, then stir well. Spoon 3 tablespoons of the sauce over the meatloaf and bake for 15 minutes. Spoon another 3 tablespoons of sauce over the meatloaf, reduce the oven temperature to 190°C (375°F/Gas 5) and bake for 1 hour 10 minutes, basting occasionally with sauce. Slice and serve with any remaining sauce and a mixed-leaf salad.

nutrition per serve Energy 1132 kJ (271 Cal); Fat 8.5 g; Saturated fat 2.9 g; Protein 23.9 g; Carbohydrate 21.6 g; Fibre 5 g; Cholesterol 74 mg; Sodium 355 mg

VEGETARIAN MEALS

THIS COLOURFUL DISH MAKES A
GREAT VEGETARIAN STARTER OR
CELEBRATORY MEAL. IF PREPARING
AS A MAIN MEAL, SERVE WITH A
DOLLOP OF YOGHURT OR SOME
CHEESE FOR EXTRA CALCIUM
AND PROTEIN.

nutrition per serve: Energy 912 kJ (218 Cal)
Fat 7.4 g
Saturated fat 2.3 g
Protein 8.9 g
Carbohydrate 26 g
Fibre 5.4 g
Cholesterol 8 mg
Sodium 366 mg

VEGETABLE AND POLENTA PIE

330 ml (11¼ fl oz/1⅓ cups) reduced-salt vegetable stock
150 g (5½ oz/1 cup) coarse polenta
50 g (1¾ oz/½ cup) finely grated parmesan cheese
1 tbsp olive oil
1 large onion, chopped
2 garlic cloves, crushed
2 eggplants (aubergines)
1 large red capsicum (pepper), diced
2 zucchini (courgettes), thickly sliced

150 g (5½ oz) button mushrooms, cut into quarters
400 g (14 oz) tin reduced-salt diced tomatoes
3 tsp balsamic vinegar
olive oil, for brushing

PREP TIME: 25 MINUTES + REFRIGERATION
COOKING TIME: 50 MINUTES
SERVES 6

Line a 22 cm (8½ in) round cake tin with foil. Pour the stock and 350 ml (12 fl oz) water into a saucepan and bring to the boil. Add the polenta in a thin stream and stir over low heat for 5 minutes, or until the liquid is absorbed and the mixture is thick and comes away from the side of the pan. Remove the pan from the heat and stir in the cheese until it melts all through the polenta. Spread into the tin, smoothing the surface as much as possible. Refrigerate until set.

Preheat the oven to 200°C (400°F/Gas 6). Heat the oil in a large saucepan and add the onion. Cook over medium heat, stirring occasionally, for 3 minutes, or until soft. Add the garlic and cook for 1 minute. Add the eggplant, capsicum, zucchini, mushrooms and tomatoes. Bring to the boil, then reduce the heat and simmer, covered, for 20 minutes, or until the vegetables are tender. Stir occasionally. Stir in the vinegar, then season with freshly ground black pepper.

Transfer the vegetable mixture to a 22 cm (8½ in) pie dish, piling it up slightly in the centre.

When the polenta has set, turn it out of the pan, peel off the foil and cut into 12 wedges. Arrange, smooth side down, in a single layer, over the vegetables—don't worry about any gaps. Brush lightly with olive oil and bake for 20 minutes, or until lightly brown and crisp.

MIDDLE-EASTERN POTATO CASEROLE

THIS DELICIOUS DISH IS EASY TO PUT TOGETHER AND EVEN EASIER TO EAT. IT'S A LOVELY MEAL TO SHARE WITH FRIENDS.

¼ tsp saffron threads

1 kg (2 lb 4 oz) potatoes, cut into large cubes

1 tsp olive oil

1 small onion, sliced

½ tsp ground turmeric

½ tsp ground coriander

250 ml (9 fl oz/1 cup) reduced-salt vegetable stock

1 garlic clove, crushed

30 g (1 oz/¼ cup) raisins

1 tsp chopped flat-leaf (Italian) parsley

1 tsp chopped coriander (cilantro) leaves

PREP TIME: 10 MINUTES

TOTAL COOKING TIME: 35 MINUTES

SERVES 4

Soak the saffron in 1 tablespoon of hot water. Put the potatoes in a saucepan of cold, salted water. Bring to the boil and cook until tender but still firm. Drain and set aside.

Heat the oil in a separate saucepan, add the onion, turmeric and ground coriander and cook over low heat for 5 minutes, or until the onion is soft.

Add the potato, vegetable stock and garlic. Bring to the boil, then reduce the heat and simmer for 10 minutes.

Add the saffron with its soaking water and the raisins, and cook for 10 minutes, or until the potato is soft and the sauce has reduced and thickened. Stir in the parsley and coriander.

HINT:
• This dish is delicious served with couscous.

nutrition per serve: Energy 919 kJ (219 Cal); Fat 1.8 g; Saturated fat 0.3 g; Protein 6.7 g; Carbohydrate 40.8 g; Fibre 5.1 g; Cholesterol 0 mg; Sodium 271 mg

MOROCCAN VEGETABLE TAGINE WITH COUSCOUS

THIS EXOTIC MIDDLE-EASTERN DISH PROVIDES A SATISFYING ALTERNATIVE TO RICE AND PASTA DISHES.

2 tsp oil
2 onions, chopped
1 tsp ground ginger
2 tsp ground paprika
2 tsp ground cumin
1 cinnamon stick
pinch of saffron threads
1.5 kg (3 lb 5 oz) mixed vegetables, peeled, and cut into large chunks (carrot, eggplant (aubergine), orange sweet potato, parsnip, potato, pumpkin (winter squash))
½ preserved lemon, rinsed, pith and flesh removed, thinly sliced
400 g (14 oz) tin reduced-salt peeled tomatoes

250 ml (9 fl oz/1 cup) reduced-salt vegetable stock
100 g (3½ oz) dried pears, halved
60 g (2¼ oz) pitted prunes
2 zucchini (courgettes), cut into large chunks
300 g (10½ oz) instant couscous
1 tbsp olive oil
3 tbsp chopped flat-leaf (Italian) parsley
50 g (1¾ oz/⅓ cup) almonds

PREP TIME: 25 MINUTES

TOTAL COOKING TIME: 1 HOUR

SERVES 4–6

Preheat the oven to 180°C (350°F/Gas 4). Heat the oil in a large saucepan or ovenproof dish, add the onion and cook over medium heat for 5 minutes, or until soft. Add the spices and cook for 3 minutes.

Add the vegetables and cook, stirring, until coated with the spices and the outsides begin to soften. Add the lemon, tomatoes, stock, pears and prunes. Cover, transfer to the oven and cook for 30 minutes. Add the zucchini and cook for 15–20 minutes, or until the vegetables are tender.

Cover the couscous with the olive oil and 500 ml (17 fl oz/2 cups) boiling water, cover and leave until all the water has been absorbed. Fluff with a fork.

Remove the cinnamon stick from the vegetables, then stir in the parsley. Serve on a large platter with the couscous formed in a ring and the vegetable tagine in the centre, sprinkle with almonds.

nutrition per serve (6): Energy 1929 kJ (461 Cal); Fat 7.7 g; Saturated fat 0.8 g; Protein 14.3 g; Carbohydrate 78.4 g; Fibre 10.6 g; Cholesterol 0 mg; Sodium 283 mg

HARISSA WITH VEGETABLE COUSCOUS

HARISSA

3 dried bird's eye chillies

3 large garlic cloves

1 tsp coriander seeds

½ tsp ground cumin

60 ml (2 fl oz/¼ cup) reduced-salt tomato
　passata (puréed tomatoes)

1 tbsp extra virgin olive oil

1 tbsp no-added-salt tomato paste
　(concentrated purée)

2 tbsp roughly chopped coriander
　(cilantro) leaves

2 tbsp roughly chopped mint

250 g (9 oz/1 cup) Greek-style
　low-fat yoghurt

300 g (10½ oz/1⅔ cups) couscous

2 tsp olive oil

1 large onion, halved and thinly sliced

3 zucchini (courgettes), thinly sliced

2 large carrots, cut into fine matchsticks
　2 cm (¾ in) long

400 g (14 oz) tin chickpeas, rinsed
　and drained

40 g (1½ oz/⅓ cup) sultanas
　(golden raisins)

30 g (1 oz/¼ cup) toasted slivered almonds

2 tbsp baby capers, rinsed and
　squeezed dry

PREP TIME: 20 MINUTES

COOKING TIME: 10 MINUTES

SERVES 4–6

To make the harissa, put the chillies, garlic, coriander seeds and cumin in a mini processor or blender. Blend for 30 seconds, or until roughly ground. Add the tomato passata, olive oil and tomato paste and blend for 12–15 seconds, or until smooth.

Put the coriander, mint and yoghurt in a small bowl and mix to combine.

Prepare the couscous according to the manufacturer's instructions. Cover and set aside. Heat the oil in a large frying pan over medium heat. Add the onion and fry for 5–6 minutes, or until softened. Add the zucchini and carrot and fry for 5 minutes, or until just tender and beginning to brown. Stir in the chickpeas and sultanas. Add the couscous, stirring gently until well combined.

Divide the couscous mixture among serving plates and sprinkle with the toasted almonds and capers. Serve accompanied by the harissa and herbed yoghurt, to be added as desired.

HINT:
• Store the harissa, covered with a thin layer of olive oil in an airtight container, in the refrigerator for 7–10 days.

THIS COLOURFUL DISH IS
A GREAT WAY TO INCLUDE
LEGUMES IN YOUR DIET, WHICH
CONTAIN PROTEIN, CALCIUM
AND GOOD AMOUNTS OF IRON.

nutrition per serve: Energy 1589 kJ (380 Cal)
Fat 8.7 g
Saturated fat 1.1 g
Protein 14.5 g
Carbohydrate 57.4 g
Fibre 6.2 g
Cholesterol 2 mg
Sodium 195 mg

CHICKPEA CURRY

THIS MILD BUT FLAVOURSOME CURRY IS SURE TO SATISFY, BUT YOU NEED TO PLAN IN ADVANCE SO THAT THE CHICKPEAS CAN SOAK OVERNIGHT.

220 g (7¾ oz/1 cup) dried chickpeas
2 tsp oil
2 onions, finely chopped
2 large tomatoes, chopped
½ tsp ground coriander
1 tsp ground cumin
1 tsp chilli powder
¼ tsp ground turmeric
1 tsp channa masala (see Hint)

1 small white onion, sliced, extra, to serve
mint and coriander (cilantro) leaves,
   to garnish
boiled rice, to serve (optional)

PREP TIME: 15 MINUTES + OVERNIGHT
   SOAKING
TOTAL COOKING TIME: 1 HOUR 15 MINUTES
SERVES 6

Put the chickpeas in a bowl, cover with water and leave to soak overnight. Drain, rinse, and put in a large saucepan. Cover with plenty of water and bring to the boil, then reduce the heat and simmer for 40 minutes, or until soft. Drain.

Heat the oil in a large saucepan, add the onion and cook over medium heat for 15 minutes, or until golden brown. Add the tomato, ground coriander and cumin, chilli powder, turmeric and channa masala, and 500 ml (16 fl oz/2 cups) water and cook for 10 minutes, or until the tomato is soft. Add the chickpeas, season with freshly ground pepper and cook for 7–10 minutes, or until the sauce thickens. Garnish with sliced onion and fresh mint and coriander leaves, and seve with rice.

HINT:
• Channa (chole) masala is a spice blend available at Indian food stores. Garam masala can be used as a substitute but the flavour will be a little different.

nutrition per serve: Energy 735 kJ (176 Cal); Fat 4 g; Saturated fat 0.5 g; Protein 8.5 g; Carbohydrate 20 g; Fibre 8.1 g; Cholesterol 0 mg; Sodium 22 mg

WILD RICE WITH PUMPKIN

THIS TASTY DISH IS RELATIVELY EASY TO COOK. WILD RICE IS MUCH HIGHER IN PROTEIN THAN REGULAR RICE AND IS ALSO A GOOD SOURCE OF NIACIN.

190 g (6¾ oz/1 cup) wild rice, rinsed

300 g (10½ oz) jap or kent pumpkin, skin on, cut into 1 x 6 cm (½ x 2½ in) wedges

400 g (14 oz) tinned chickpeas, drained and rinsed

8 spring onions (scallions), finely sliced

50 g (1¾ oz/⅓ cup) currants

70 g (2½ oz/½ cup) pistachio nuts, roughly chopped

1 tsp garam masala

3 tbsp pepitas (pumpkin seeds)

1 tbsp olive oil

2 tsp finely grated orange zest

1 large handful coriander (cilantro) leaves

1 large handful mint, torn

PREP TIME: 20 MINUTES

COOKING TIME: 40 MINUTES

SERVES 4–6

Put the rice in a small saucepan over medium–high heat, add 625 ml (21½ fl oz/ 2½ cups) water and cover with a lid. Bring to the boil, then reduce the heat to low and simmer for 30–35 minutes, or until all of the liquid has been absorbed and the rice is cooked but still *al dente*.

Line a steamer with baking paper and punch with holes. Arrange the pumpkin on top and cover with a lid. Sit the steamer over a saucepan or wok of boiling water and steam for 5 minutes, or until the pumpkin is tender when pierced with a sharp knife. Set aside to cool a little.

Put the chickpeas, spring onion, currants, pistachios, garam masala, pepitas, oil, orange zest, coriander and mint leaves in a large bowl and season with freshly ground black pepper. Add the steamed rice and pumpkin wedges and toss gently to combine. Arrange the salad in a bowl or on a platter and serve warm.

nutrition per serve (6): Energy 1296 kJ (310 Cal); Fat 13 g; Saturated fat 1.8 g; Protein 11.2 g; Carbohydrate 34.2 g; Fibre 6.7 g; Cholesterol 0 mg; Sodium 113 mg

THIS SPICY DISH CONTAINS
EGGPLANT, WHICH IS A GREAT
VEGETABLE TO INCLUDE IN A
LOW-CHOLESTEROL DIET. IT
IS LOW IN FAT AND SODIUM
AND IS CHOLESTEROL FREE.

nutrition per serve: Energy 1310 kJ (313 Cal)
Fat 5.7 g
Saturated fat 0.7 g
Protein 7.6 g
Carbohydrate 53.2 g
Fibre 5.1 g
Cholesterol 0 mg
Sodium 24 mg

140

CURRIED EGGPLANT STIR-FRY

1 tbsp vegetable oil
½–1 long green chilli, finely sliced
4 red Asian shallots, chopped
2 garlic cloves, finely sliced
2–3 tsp curry powder, to taste
350 g (12 oz) slender eggplants
 (aubergines), cut on the diagonal into
 1 cm (½ in) slices
3 vine-ripened tomatoes, each cut into
 8 wedges

70 g (2½ oz/1½ cups) baby English
 spinach leaves
boiled basmati rice, to serve

PREP TIME: 15 MINUTES

COOKING TIME: 15 MINUTES

SERVES 4

Heat the oil in a large wok and swirl to coat. Add the green chilli, shallots and garlic and stir-fry over high heat for 1 minute. Stir in the curry powder and stir-fry for 1 minute.

Add the eggplant and stir-fry for 3 minutes, or until the eggplant has softened a little. Add the tomato and 125 ml (4 fl oz/½ cup) water. Cover the wok and cook for 10 minutes, or until the eggplant is cooked, stirring occasionally. Stir in the spinach leaves and cook for 1 minute, or until wilted. Serve immediately with boiled rice.

CHILLI TOFU STIR-FRY

TOFU IS A GREAT INGREDIENT TO CARRY FLAVOURS, SOAKING UP THE
COOKING JUICES IN A DISH. IT IS HIGH IN PROTEIN AND CONTAINS SOME IRON.

1 tbsp canola oil
1 tsp bottled crushed chilli
2 tsp grated fresh ginger
2 garlic cloves, crushed
250 g (9 oz) firm tofu, cut into 1.5 cm
  (^{5}/$_8$ in) cubes
8 spring onions (scallions), sliced on the
  diagonal
150 g (5^1/$_2$ oz) fresh baby corn, halved
  lengthways
150 g (5^1/$_2$ oz) snowpeas (mangetout),
  topped and tailed

500 g (1 lb 2 oz) hokkien (egg) noodles
40 g (1^1/$_2$ oz/^{1}/$_4$ cup) cashew nuts
1 tbsp reduced-sodium soy sauce
125 ml (4 fl oz/^{1}/$_2$ cup) reduced-salt
  vegetable stock
1 handful coriander (cilantro) leaves

PREP TIME: 15 MINUTES
COOKING TIME: 15 MINUTES
SERVES 4

Heat the oil in a wok over medium heat and swirl to coat. Add the chilli, ginger and garlic
and stir-fry for about 2–3 minutes, or until aromatic. Add the tofu cubes, spring onion and
baby corn and stir-fry for 2–3 minutes.

Add the snowpeas, noodles and cashews and cook, stirring, for 3–5 minutes, or until the
vegetables are almost tender. Stir in the soy sauce and stock, then bring to the boil and
simmer for 2 minutes, or until slightly reduced. Stir in the coriander and serve immediately.

nutrition per serve: Energy 1596 kJ (381 Cal); Fat 15.5 g; Saturated fat 2.1 g; Protein 16.8 g;
Carbohydrate 41.1 g; Fibre 7.3 g; Cholesterol 0 mg; Sodium 524 mg

PUMPKIN BHAJI

BHAJIS ARE POPULAR INDIAN VEGETABLE DISHES. THIS ONE IS MADE WITH PUMPKIN, WHICH CONTAINS VITAMIN A AND ANTIOXIDANT CAROTENOIDS, PARTICULARLY ALPHA- AND BETA-CAROTENES.

1 tbsp vegetable oil
1 tsp yellow mustard seeds
1 onion, finely chopped
1 tsp grated fresh ginger
1 green chilli, seeded and chopped
1 tsp ground coriander
$\frac{1}{2}$ tsp garam masala
$\frac{1}{2}$ tsp ground turmeric
$\frac{1}{2}$ tsp ground cumin
$\frac{1}{2}$ tsp chilli flakes

750 g (1 lb 10 oz) pumpkin (winter squash), peeled, seeded and cut into 3 cm (1$\frac{1}{4}$ in) cubes
400 g (14 oz) tin reduced-salt diced tomatoes
1 tsp soft brown sugar
3 tbsp low-fat plain yoghurt
coriander (cilantro) leaves, to serve
boiled basmati rice, to serve

PREP TIME: 20 MINUTES
COOKING TIME: 35 MINUTES
SERVES 4

Heat the oil in a large wok and cook the mustard seeds until they just start to pop. Add the onion, ginger and chilli and stir-fry for 2 minutes. Add the coriander, garam masala, turmeric, cumin and chilli flakes and stir-fry for 1 minute, or until aromatic.

Stir in the pumpkin, chopped tomatoes, sugar and 125 ml (4 fl oz/$\frac{1}{2}$ cup) water. Bring to the boil, then reduce the heat and simmer, covered, for 30 minutes, or until the pumpkin is tender. Stir occasionally. Gently fold in the yoghurt and scatter with coriander leaves before serving with boiled rice.

nutrition per serve: Energy 1608 kJ (384 Cal); Fat 6.5 g; Saturated fat 1.3 g; Protein 10.8 g; Carbohydrate 66 g; Fibre 5 g; Cholesterol 1 mg; Sodium 37 mg

ASIAN GREENS WITH CHILLI AND COCONUT MARINADE

MARINADE
15 g (½ oz/¼ cup) shredded coconut
2 garlic cloves, roughly chopped
2 cm (¾ in) piece ginger, roughly chopped
1 red Asian shallot, roughly chopped
1 small red chilli, sliced
2 tbsp canola oil
1 tbsp rice vinegar
2 tsp fish sauce
1 tsp soft brown sugar
2 spring onions (scallions), sliced

1.1 kg (2 lb 7 oz/2 bunches) Asian green vegetables
boiled rice, to serve (optional)

PREP TIME: 25 MINUTES + 1 HOUR MARINATING
COOKING TIME: 10 MINUTES
SERVES 4

To make the marinade, heat a dry frying pan over medium heat. Add the shredded coconut and fry, stirring, for 3–4 minutes, or until brown. Transfer the coconut to a spice mill or mini processor, add the garlic, ginger, shallot and chilli and blend until finely chopped. Add 1 tablespoon of oil, vinegar, fish sauce and sugar and blend in short bursts until blended. Transfer to a large bowl and stir in the spring onion.

Slice the Asian green vegetables into 8 cm (3¼ in) lengths and divide these into stems and leaves. Heat a wok or large frying pan over medium–high heat and add the remaining oil. Add the vegetable stems and stir-fry for 1 minute. Add the vegetable leaves and stir-fry for 45–60 seconds, or until they wilt and turn bright green.

Transfer the hot vegetables to the bowl with the marinade and toss to coat. Marinate for at least 1 hour to allow the flavours to develop.

Serve the vegetables with the boiled rice.

TRY THIS TASTY DISH, COMBINING THE NUTRITIOUS GOODNESS OF GREENS WITH THE FLAVOUR BURST OF CHILLI AND FRESH COCONUT.

nutrition per serve: Energy 934 kJ (223 Cal)
Fat 19.8 g
Saturated fat 4.3 g
Protein 4.1 g
Carbohydrate 5.2 g
Fibre 5.1 g
Cholesterol 0 mg
Sodium 265 mg

PASTA SIRACUSA

THIS MEDITERRANEAN-STYLE DISH IS A GOOD SOURCE OF ANTIOXIDANTS. IF YOU'RE WATCHING YOUR WEIGHT USE WHOLEMEAL SPAGHETTI BECAUSE IT IS MORE FILLING THAN WHITE PASTA.

2 tsp olive oil

2 garlic cloves, crushed

1 large green capsicum (pepper),
   thinly sliced

2 x 400 g (14 oz) tins reduced-salt diced
   tomatoes

2 zucchini (courgettes), chopped

2 anchovy fillets in brine, drained
   and chopped

1 tbsp capers, chopped

3 tbsp black olives in brine, rinsed, pitted
   and halved

2 tbsp chopped basil

500 g (1 lb 2 oz) spaghetti or linguine

65 g (1¼ oz/⅓ oz/⅔ cup) grated parmesan
   cheese, to serve

PREP TIME: 20 MINUTES

COOKING TIME: 30 MINUTES

SERVES 4–6

Heat the oil in a large, deep frying pan and cook the garlic for 30 seconds over low heat. Add the capsicum, tomatoes, zucchini, anchovies, capers, olives and 125 ml (4 fl oz/ ½ cup) water. Cook for 20 minutes, stirring occasionally.

Add the basil to the pan and stir well. Season to taste with freshly ground black pepper.

Meanwhile, cook the pasta in a large saucepan of boiling water for 10 minutes, or until al dente. Drain well. Serve the pasta topped with the sauce and grated parmesan.

nutrition per serve (6): Energy 1651 kJ (394 Cal); Fat 6.5 g; Saturated fat 2.7 g; Protein 15.7 g; Carbohydrate 64.5 g; Fibre 5.4 g; Cholesterol 11 mg; Sodium 260 mg

SPINACH SHELLS IN TOMATO SAUCE

THIS LOW-FAT MEAL IS SUITABLE FOR VEGETARIANS WHO EAT DAIRY PRODUCTS AND IT PROVIDES GOOD AMOUNTS OF CALCIUM, B-GROUP VITAMINS AND ANTIOXIDANTS.

30 (220 g/7 oz) large pasta shells
250 g (9 oz) frozen leaf spinach, defrosted
500 g (1 lb 2 oz/2 cups) low-fat, reduced-salt cottage cheese
250 g (9 oz/1 cup) low-fat ricotta cheese
2 spring onions (scallions), finely chopped
1 tsp nutmeg
500 ml (17 fl oz/2 cups) reduced-salt tomato passata (puréed tomatoes)

250 ml (9 fl oz/1 cup) reduced-salt vegetable stock or water
60 g (2¼ oz/½ cup) grated reduced-fat cheddar cheese (we used 50% reduced-fat)

PREP TIME: 20 MINUTES
COOKING TIME: 55 MINUTES
SERVES 4–6

Cook the pasta in a large saucepan of boiling salted water for 10 minutes, or until *al dente*. Drain and cool under cold water.

Using clean hands, squeeze the excess moisture from the spinach. Put in a large bowl, add the cottage and ricotta cheeses, spring onions and nutmeg. Season well with freshly ground black pepper. Combine well using a fork.

Preheat the oven to 180°C (350°F/Gas 4). Combine half the tomato passata and half the stock or water and pour over the base of a 32 x 25 x 5 cm (12½ x 10 x 2 in) ovenproof dish. Spoon the spinach mixture into the pasta shells and put them in a single layer over the sauce. Spread over the remaining passata and stock or water and sprinkle over the cheese mixture.

Bake for 45 minutes, or until the pasta is cooked. Serve hot with a mixed green salad.

HINT:
• This meal can be prepared in advance.

nutrition per serve (6): Energy 1322 kJ (316 Cal); Fat 5.8 g; Saturated fat 2.7 g; Protein 26.1 g; Carbohydrate 37.6 g; Fibre 4.9 g; Cholesterol 18 mg; Sodium 568 mg

RATATOUILLE IS A VERSATILE
DISH THAT CAN BE SERVED
WITH RICE, POTATOES OR AS
A SIDE. HERE IT IS SERVED
ACCOMPANIED BY PASTA AS A
COMPLETE VEGETARIAN MEAL.

nutrition per serve: Energy 1610 kJ (385 Cal)
Fat 5.4 g
Saturated fat 1.8 g
Protein 12.6 g
Carbohydrate 65.5 g
Fibre 6.8 g
Cholesterol 11 mg
Sodium 31 mg

CREAMY RATATOUILLE WITH FARFALLE

350 g (12 oz) baby eggplants (aubergines)
olive oil spray
1 large red capsicum (pepper)
1 large green capsicum (pepper)
2 tsp olive oil
1 onion, diced
4 garlic cloves, crushed
400 g (14 oz) tin reduced-salt diced
   tomatoes
2 zucchini (courgettes), finely diced
1 tbsp chopped thyme
3 tbsp chopped parsley
3 tbsp red wine

2 tsp soft brown sugar
2 tsp no-added-salt tomato paste
   (concentrated purée)
2½ handfuls basil, plus extra whole leaves,
   to serve
500 g (1 lb 2 oz) farfalle pasta
100 ml (3½ fl oz) extra-light pouring
   (whipping) cream

PREP TIME: 30 MINUTES
COOKING TIME: 55 MINUTES
SERVES 6

Heat the grill (broiler) to high. Cut the ends off the eggplants and slice the flesh length-ways into 2 cm (¾ in) strips. Spread the eggplant on a baking tray lined with foil and lightly spray with spray oil. Grill for about 3–5 minutes, or until golden brown, then remove.

Cut the capsicums into large flat pieces and remove the seeds and membranes. Cook, skin side up, under the hot grill until the skin blackens and blisters. Leave to cool in a plastic bag, then peel away the skin and cut the flesh into strips.

Heat the oil in a large frying pan. Add the onion and garlic and gently sauté for 3 minutes. Stir through the grilled eggplant, capsicum, tomato, zucchini, thyme, parsley, wine, sugar, tomato paste and basil. Season well with freshly ground pepper, then simmer, uncovered, for 30 minutes, stirring occasionally.

While the ratatouille is simmering, cook the pasta in a large saucepan of rapidly boiling salted water for 10 minutes, or until *al dente*. Drain well and keep warm.

Take the ratatouille off the heat, add the cream and stir through gently. Divide the pasta among six serving bowls and spoon the ratatouille over the top. Garnish with the extra basil leaves and serve.

RED LENTIL AND RICOTTA LASAGNE

THIS LOW GI LASAGNE IS AN EXCELLENT CHOICE FOR VEGETARIANS. IT
PROVIDES GOOD AMOUNTS OF COMPLETE PROTEIN, CALCIUM AND ANTIOXIDANTS.

90 g (3¼ oz/½ cup) red lentils
2 tsp olive oil
2–3 garlic cloves, crushed
1 large onion, chopped
1 small red capsicum (pepper), chopped
2 zucchini (courgettes), sliced
1 celery stalk, sliced
2 x 400 g (14 oz) tins reduced-salt diced
 tomatoes
2 tbsp no-added-salt tomato paste
 (concentrated purée)
1 tsp dried oregano
40 g (1½ oz/⅓ cup) cornflour (cornstarch)
750 ml (26 fl oz/3 cups) skim milk

¼ onion
½ tsp ground nutmeg
350 g (12 oz/1⅓ cups) low-fat ricotta
 cheese
12 dried or fresh lasagne sheets
60 g (2¼ oz/½ cup) grated reduced-fat
 cheddar cheese

PREP TIME: 30 MINUTES + 30 MINUTES
 SOAKING
COOKING TIME: 1 HOUR 50 MINUTES
SERVES 6

Pour the lentils in a large bowl, cover with boiling water and soak for 30 minutes. Drain. Heat the oil in a large saucepan, add the garlic and onion and cook for 2 minutes. Add the capsicum, zucchini and celery and cook for 2–3 minutes, or until softened. Add the lentils, tomatoes, tomato paste, oregano and 375 ml (13 fl oz/1½ cups) water. Bring slowly to the boil, then reduce the heat and simmer for 30 minutes, or until the lentils are tender. Stir occasionally. Preheat the oven to 180°C (350°F/Gas 4).

To make the white sauce, blend the cornflour with 2 tablespoons of the milk in a saucepan until smooth. Pour the remaining milk into the pan, add the onion and stir over low heat until the mixture boils and thickens. Add the nutmeg and season with freshly ground black pepper, then cook over low heat for 5 minutes. Remove the onion.

Beat the ricotta with about 125 ml (4 fl oz/½ cup) of the white sauce. Spread one-third of the lentil mixture over the base of a 3-litre (105 fl oz/12 cup) ovenproof dish. Cover with a layer of lasagne sheets. Spread another third of the lentil mixture over the pasta, then spread the ricotta mixture evenly over the top. Follow with another layer of lasagne, then the remaining lentils. Pour the white sauce over the top. Sprinkle with the grated cheese. Bake for 1 hour, covering with lightly oiled foil if the top starts to brown too much. Stand for 5 minutes before cutting. Serve with a salad.

nutrition per serve: Energy 1667 kJ (398 Cal); Fat 7.9 g; Saturated fat 2.9 g; Protein 23.7 g; Carbohydrate 55.4 g; Fibre 6.9 g; Cholesterol 10 mg; Sodium 232 mg

SPICY VEGETABLE STEW WITH DHAL

THIS INDIAN-STYLE DISH COMBINES THE GOODNESS OF FRESH VEGETABLES AND LEGUMES, PROVIDING A NOURISHING AND FILLING MEAL. IT IS LOW IN FAT, CHOLESTEROL-FREE, AND A GOOD SOURCE OF FOLATE AND POTASSIUM.

DHAL
165 g (5½ oz/¾ cup) yellow split peas
5 cm (2 in) piece of ginger, grated
2–3 garlic cloves, crushed
1 red chilli, seeded and chopped

3 tomatoes
1 tbsp oil
1 tsp yellow mustard seeds
1 tsp cumin seeds
1 tsp ground cumin
½ tsp garam masala
1 red onion, cut into thin wedges

3 slender eggplants (aubergines), thickly sliced
2 carrots, thickly sliced
¼ cauliflower, cut into florets
375 ml (12 fl oz/1½ cups) reduced-salt vegetable stock
2 small zucchini (courgettes), thickly sliced
90 g (3 oz/½ cup) frozen peas
15 g (½ oz/½ cup) fresh coriander (cilantro) leaves

PREP TIME: 25 MINUTES + 2 HOURS SOAKING
COOKING TIME: 1 HOUR 35 MINUTES
SERVES 4–6

To make the dhal, put the split peas in a bowl, cover with water and soak for 2 hours. Drain. Place in a large saucepan with the ginger, garlic, chilli and 750 ml (26 fl oz/3 cups) water. Bring to the boil, reduce the heat and simmer for 45 minutes, or until soft.

Score a cross in the base of each tomato, soak in boiling water for 30 seconds, then plunge into cold water and peel the skin away from the cross. Seed and thoroughly chop.

Heat the oil in a large saucepan. Cook the spices over medium heat for 30 seconds, or until fragrant. Add the onion and cook for 2 minutes, or until the onion is soft. Stir in the tomato, eggplant, carrot and cauliflower.

Add the dhal and stock, mix together well and simmer, covered, for 45 minutes, or until the vegetables are tender. Stir occasionally. Add the zucchini and peas during the last 10 minutes of cooking. Stir in the coriander leaves and serve.

nutrition per serve (6): Energy 746 kJ (178 Cal); Fat 4.5 g; Saturated fat 0.4 g; Protein 10 g; Carbohydrate 21.2 g; Fibre 7.3 g; Cholesterol 0 mg; Sodium 282 mg

CARAMELIZED ONIONS AND LENTILS WITH ENGLISH SPINACH

225 g (8 oz/1¼ cups) puy lentils or tiny
   blue-green lentils
1 tbsp olive oil
2 red onions, finely sliced
2 garlic cloves, finely chopped
1 tsp ground coriander
1 tsp ground cumin
550 g (1 lb 4 oz) English spinach, rinsed
   well and stems trimmed

1 tbsp lemon juice
2 tbsp chopped coriander (cilantro) leaves

PREP TIME: 20 MINUTES
COOKING TIME: 1 HOUR
SERVES 6

Put the lentils in a small saucepan over high heat and add 625 ml (21½ fl oz/2½ cups) water. Bring to the boil, then cover with a fitted lid, reduce the heat to very low and simmer the lentils for 35 minutes, or until all of the water has been absorbed and the lentils are tender.

Meanwhile, heat the oil in a frying pan over medium heat and cook the onion, stirring occasionally, for 20 minutes, or until soft and caramelized. Add the garlic, ground coriander and cumin, season with freshly ground black pepper and cook for a further 3 minutes. Remove from the heat.

Put the spinach in a large steamer and cover with a lid. Sit the steamer over a saucepan or wok of boiling water and steam for 3–5 minutes, or until wilted. Combine the lentils, onion mixture and spinach in a large bowl, add the lemon juice and coriander and toss well. Serve immediately.

THIS DELICIOUS VEGETARIAN
DISH IS LOW-GI, HIGH IN FIBRE
AND A GOOD SOURCE OF
FOLATE AND ANTIOXIDANTS.

nutrition per serve: Energy 693 kJ (166 Cal)
Fat 4.2 g
Saturated fat 0.6 g
Protein 11.8 g
Carbohydrate 16.9 g
Fibre 8.2 g
Cholesterol 0 mg
Sodium 25 mg

153

SPINACH PIE

YOU CAN STILL ENJOY DELICIOUS PIES, IN MODERATION, ON A LOW-FAT DIET—
JUST MAKE SURE THEY'RE MADE WITH FILO PASTRY AND LOW-FAT FILLINGS.

olive or canola oil spray
1.5 kg (3 lb 5 oz) English spinach, trimmed
   and washed
2 tsp olive oil
1 onion, chopped
4 spring onions, chopped
750 g (1 lb 10 oz) low-fat cottage cheese
2 eggs, lightly beaten
2 garlic cloves, crushed
pinch of ground nutmeg

15 g (½ oz/¼ cup) chopped mint
8 sheets filo pastry
40 g (1½ oz/½ cup) fresh breadcrumbs

PREP TIME: 25 MINUTES
COOKING TIME: 50 MINUTES
SERVES 6

Preheat the oven to 180°C (350°F/Gas 4). Lightly spray a 24 cm square x 5 cm deep
(1.5 litre/52 fl oz/6 cups) ovenproof dish with oil. Place the spinach in a large pan. Cover
and cook for 2–3 minutes, or until just wilted. Drain, cool, then squeeze dry and chop.

Heat the oil in a small frying pan. Cook the onion and spring onion for 2–3 minutes, or until
softened. Combine with the spinach. Stir in the cheese, egg, garlic, nutmeg and mint.
Season with freshly ground black pepper, and mix thoroughly.

Spray a sheet of filo pastry with spray oil. Fold in half widthways and line the base and
sides of the dish. Repeat with three more sheets. Keep the unused sheets moist by
covering with a damp tea towel (dish towel).

Sprinkle the breadcrumbs over the pastry. Spread the filling in the dish. Fold over any
overlapping pastry. Spray and fold another sheet and place on top. Repeat with three
more sheets. Tuck the pastry in. Spray the top with more oil. Score squares on top. Bake
for 40 minutes, or until golden.

nutrition per serve: Energy 1233 kJ (295 Cal); Fat 7.1 g; Saturated fat 2 g; Protein 33.2 g;
Carbohydrate 20.2 g; Fibre 7.9 g; Cholesterol 79 mg; Sodium 416 mg

BAKED VEGETABLES WITH GARLIC AND ROSEMARY

WITH LESS FAT THAN REGULAR ROAST VEGETABLES, THIS HEALTHY COMBINATION PROVIDES CARBOHYDRATE ENERGY, FIBRE, BETA-CAROTENE, FOLATE AND POTASSIUM.

2 carrots

2 parsnips

2 large potatoes

300 g (10½ oz) pumpkin (winter squash)

olive oil spray

2 finger eggplants (aubergines)

4 large garlic cloves, unpeeled

4 small sprigs of rosemary

2 tbsp chopped parsley

PREP TIME: 15 MINUTES

COOKING TIME: 40 MINUTES

SERVES 4

Preheat the oven to 200°C (400°F/Gas 6). Wash the vegetables and pat dry. Cut the carrots and parsnips in half lengthways, then crossways. Quarter the potatoes. Cut the unpeeled pumpkin into chunks.

Put the carrot, parsnip, potato and pumpkin in a baking dish and spray lightly with oil. Sprinkle with freshly ground black pepper. Bake for 20 minutes, turning occasionally.

Meanwhile, cut the eggplants in half lengthways and make thin shallow cuts through the skin. Add to the baking dish with the garlic and rosemary sprigs. Spray with more oil and cook, turning occasionally, for 20 minutes, or until all of the vegetables are tender. To serve, squeeze out the soft garlic and serve with the vegetables and the rosemary. Sprinkle with the parsley and more freshly ground black pepper.

nutrition per serve: Energy 640 kJ (153 Cal); Fat 1.9 g; Saturated fat 0.4 g; Protein 5.4 g; Carbohydrate 24.8 g; Fibre 6 g; Cholesterol 0 mg; Sodium 30 mg

YOU'LL GET ALL YOUR NUTRIENTS IN ONE HIT WITH THIS SPICY VEGETARIAN BURGER. MUCH BETTER THAN TAKE-AWAY AND TASTIER TOO!

nutrition per serve: Energy 1530 kJ (365 Cal)
Fat 6.1 g
Saturated fat 1.2 g
Protein 15.3 g
Carbohydrate 56.6 g
Fibre 9.2 g
Cholesterol 3 mg
Sodium 395 mg

CHICKPEA BURGERS

CHICKPEA PATTIES
2 tsp olive oil
1 small onion, finely chopped
2 garlic cloves, crushed
800 g (28 oz) tinned chickpeas, drained
    and rinsed
95 g (3½ oz/½ cup) cooked brown rice
50 g (1¾ oz/⅓ cup) sun-dried tomatoes,
    chopped

1 eggplant (aubergine), cut into 1 cm
    (½ in) slices
1 large red onion, sliced into rings
spray olive oil

2 large handfuls rocket (arugula) leaves
6 pieces Turkish bread

SPICY YOGHURT DRESSING
200 g (7 oz) reduced-fat plain yoghurt
1 garlic clove, crushed
¼ tsp ground cumin
¼ tsp ground coriander

PREP TIME: 30 MINUTES + 1 HOUR
    REFRIGERATION
COOKING TIME: 20 MINUTES
MAKES 6

To make the chickpea patties, heat the oil in a frying pan and cook the onion over medium heat for 2 minutes, or until soft and lightly golden. Add the garlic and cook for 1 more minute, then remove from the heat and allow to cool slightly. Put the onion mixture in a food processor or blender with the chickpeas, rice and sun-dried tomato. Using a pulse action, process in short bursts until the mixture is combined and the chickpeas are broken up, but not completely mushy, scraping the bowl down with a spatula a few times during processing. Season with freshly ground black pepper, then shape the mixture into six patties about 8 cm (3¼ in) in diameter. Place on a tray lined with plastic wrap, then cover and refrigerate for 1 hour.

Put all the spicy yoghurt dressing ingredients in a small bowl and mix together well. Refrigerate until needed.

Preheat a barbecue hot plate to moderately hot. Spray the eggplant slices and onion rings lightly on each side with spray oil. Cook the eggplant and onion on the hotplate until tender and lightly golden—the eggplant will need about 3–4 minutes each side, the onion about 5 minutes. Transfer the vegetables to a plate and set aside.

Spray the top of the chickpea patties lightly with oil, then put them face-down on the hotplate and cook for 3 minutes. Spray the top of the patties with a little more oil, then turn and cook for a further 3 minutes, or until golden.

While the chickpea patties are cooking, arrange the rocket, barbecued eggplant and onion on the Turkish bread slices. Add the hot chickpea patties, dollop with some of the spicy yoghurt dressing and serve at once.

VEGETABLE FRITTATA

A NOURISHING SNACK OR MEAL WITH MORE NUTRIENTS THAN SCRAMBLED EGGS, THIS DISH IS A GOOD SOURCE OF VITAMIN A, FOLATE, VITAMIN B12 AND HIGH-QUALITY PROTEIN.

200 g (7 oz) zucchini (courgettes), cubed
250 g (9 oz) pumpkin (winter squash), cubed
300 g (10½ oz) potato, cubed
100 g (3½ oz) broccoli florets
2 tsp olive oil
1 small onion, chopped
1 small red capsicum (pepper), chopped

2 tbsp finely chopped fresh parsley
olive oil spray
3 eggs
2 egg whites
mixed-leaf salad, to serve

PREP TIME: 25 MINUTES
COOKING TIME: 25 MINUTES
SERVES 6

Steam the zucchini, pumpkin, potato and broccoli until tender, then transfer to a bowl.

Heat the oil in a non-stick frying pan, about 22 cm (8½ in) in diameter. Add the onion and capsicum, and cook for 3 minutes, or until tender. Transfer to the bowl of steamed vegetables, along with the chopped parsley.

Heat a frying pan over medium heat and spray with oil. Return all the vegetables to the pan and spread out with a spatula to an even thickness. Beat the eggs and egg whites together and pour into the pan, tilting to distribute evenly.

Cook over medium heat until the egg is almost set, but still runny on top. Wrap the handle of the pan in a damp tea towel (dish towel) to protect it and place the pan under the grill to cook the frittata top (pierce gently with a fork to make sure it is cooked through). Cut into wedges and serve.

nutrition per serve: Energy 542 kJ (129 Cal); Fat 5.2 g; Saturated fat 1.2 g; Protein 8 g; Carbohydrate 11.1 g; Fibre 3 g; Cholesterol 94 mg; Sodium 59 mg

SILVERBEET PARCELS

A DELICIOUS BLEND OF RISOTTO, CHEESE AND VEGETABLES IN NUTRITIOUS
SILVERBEET DELIVERS CARBOHYDRATE, B-GROUP VITAMINS, FOLATE, VITAMIN C
AND POTASSIUM.

500 ml (17 fl oz/2 cups) reduced-salt
   vegetable stock
2 tsp olive oil
1 onion, chopped
2 garlic cloves, crushed
110 g (3¾ oz/½ cup) arborio rice
1 red capsicum (pepper), chopped
250 g (9 oz) mushrooms, chopped
60 g (2¼ oz/½ cup) reduced-fat cheddar
   cheese, grated

15 g (½ oz/¼ cup) shredded fresh basil
6 large silverbeet leaves
2 x 400 g (14 oz) tins reduced-salt diced
   tomatoes
1 tbsp balsamic vinegar
1 tsp soft brown sugar

PREP TIME: 40 MINUTES
COOKING TIME: 1 HOUR
SERVES 6

Heat the stock in a pan and maintain at simmering point. Heat the oil in a large pan, add the onion and garlic and cook until softened. Add the rice, capsicum and mushrooms, and stir until well combined. Gradually add 125 ml (4 fl oz/½ cup) hot stock, stirring until the liquid is absorbed. Add the stock, a little at a time, stirring until it is all absorbed and the rice is tender (about 20 minutes). Remove from the heat, add the cheese and basil, and season well with freshly ground black pepper.

Meanwhile, trim the stalks from the silverbeet and cook the leaves, a few at a time, in a large pan of boiling water for 30 seconds, or until wilted. Drain on a tea towel (dish towel). Cut away any tough white veins from the leaves. Put a portion of risotto filling in the centre of each leaf, fold in the sides and roll up carefully. Tie with string.

Put the tomato, vinegar and sugar in a large, deep non-stick frying pan and stir to combine. Add the silverbeet parcels, cover and simmer for 10 minutes. Remove the string and serve with tomato sauce.

nutrition per serve: Energy 781 kJ (187 Cal); Fat 4.5 g; Saturated fat 1.6 g; Protein 9 g; Carbohydrate 24.2 g; Fibre 6.1 g; Cholesterol 6 mg; Sodium 420 mg

SWEET POTATO STRUDEL

250 g (9 oz) orange sweet potato, cut into
  2 cm (¾ in) cubes
3 garlic cloves, unpeeled
olive oil spray
250 g (9 oz) English spinach, blanched and
  excess moisture squeezed out, roughly
  chopped
40 g (1½ oz/¼ cup) pine nuts, toasted
125 g (4½ oz) low-fat feta cheese, crumbled
3 spring onions (scallions), including green
  part, chopped

50 g (1 ¾ oz) black olives, pitted and sliced
15 g (½ oz/¼ cup) chopped basil
1 tbsp chopped rosemary
8 sheets filo pastry
1 tbsp sesame seeds

PREP TIME: 25 MINUTES

COOKING TIME: 1 HOUR 5 MINUTES

SERVES 6

Preheat the oven to moderate 180°C (350°F/Gas 4). Put the sweet potato and garlic in a roasting tin and spray with oil. Roast for 30 minutes, or until the sweet potato is soft. Remove the garlic when it is soft, after about 15 minutes. Cool slightly.

Combine the sweet potato, spinach, pine nuts, feta, spring onion, olives, basil and rosemary. Peel the garlic cloves and roughly chop the flesh, then add to the sweet potato mixture, and season with freshly ground black pepper.

Cover the pastry with a damp tea towel (dish towel) to prevent it drying out. Lay the pastry out in front of you, in a stack, and spray each layer with oil. Spread the filling in the centre of the pastry, covering an area 10 x 30 cm. Fold in the shorter ends of the pastry. Fold the long side closest to you over the filling, then carefully roll up. Place the strudel on a greased baking tray, seam side down. Spray with oil and sprinkle with sesame seeds. Bake for 35 minutes, or until crisp and golden. Serve warm.

THIS TASTY AND COLOURFUL DISH
IS GREAT TO SERVE TO FRIENDS.
THE VARIETY OF INGREDIENTS
DELIVERS GOOD AMOUNTS
OF MONOUNSATURATED FAT
AND FIBRE.

nutrition per serve: Energy 925 kJ (221 Cal)
Fat 10.9 g
Saturated fat 2.6 g
Protein 9.9 g
Carbohydrate 19.1 g
Fibre 3.6 g
Cholesterol 4 mg
Sodium 436 mg

161

SWEET THINGS

MANGO PASSIONFRUIT SORBET

CLEBRATE THE SUMMER MONTHS WITH THIS TASTY SORBET. IT CONTAINS GOOD AMOUNTS OF FIBRE AND ANTIOXIDANTS.

**230 g (8 ½ oz/1 cup) caster
  (superfine) sugar
90 g (3¼ oz/⅓ cup) passionfruit pulp
  (about 8 passionfruit)
½ large mango, chopped
1 large peach, chopped
2 tbsp lemon juice
1 egg white**

PREP TIME: 20 MINUTES + REFRIGERATION
  TIME + 8 HOURS FREEZING
COOKING TIME: 5 MINUTES
SERVES 6

Put the sugar in a saucepan with 250 ml (9 fl oz/1 cup) water. Stir over low heat until the sugar has dissolved. Increase the heat, bring to the boil and boil for 1 minute. Transfer to a glass bowl, cool, then refrigerate. Strain the passionfruit pulp, reserving 1 tablespoon of the seeds.

Blend the fruit, passionfruit juice and lemon juice in a blender until smooth. With the motor running, add the cold sugar syrup and 150 ml (5 fl oz) water. Stir in the passionfruit seeds. Freeze in a shallow container, stirring occasionally, for about 5 hours, or until almost set.

Break up the icy mixture roughly with a fork or spoon, transfer to a bowl and beat with electric beaters until smooth and fluffy. Beat the egg white in a small bowl until firm peaks form, then fold into the mixture until just combined. Spread into a loaf tin and return to the freezer until firm. Transfer to the refrigerator, to soften, 15 minutes before serving.

HINT:
• To make a berry sorbet, use 200 g (7 oz) blackberries or blueberries, 200 g (7 oz) hulled
  strawberries and 50 g (1¾ oz) peach flesh. Prepare as above.

nutrition per serve: Energy 788 kJ (188 Cal); Fat 0.1 g; Saturated fat 0 g; Protein 1.6 g;
Carbohydrate 44.7 g; Fibre 3 g; Cholesterol 0 mg; Sodium 13 mg

PEAR SORBET

THIS FRESH FRUIT SORBET IS MADE WITH SUCRALOSE INSTEAD OF SUGAR SO IT'S GOOD IF YOU ARE WATCHING YOUR WEIGHT OR HAVE DIABETES.

6 large (2 kg/4 lb 8 oz) very ripe pears
25 g (1 oz/1 cup) sucralose

PREP TIME: 40 MINUTES + OVERNIGHT FREEZING
COOKING TIME: 15 MINUTES
SERVES 4–6

Thickly peel the pears, then core them and slice them into thick pieces. Place the pears in a large saucepan, just cover with water and simmer for about 10 minutes, or until tender. Drain and allow to cool.

Purée the pears in a blender or food processor until smooth.

Combine the sucralose and 200 ml (7 fl oz) water in a saucepan over medium heat. Allow the syrup to cool. Mix together the sucralose syrup and pear purée, then pour into a shallow metal pan. Freeze until just solid.

Remove the pan from the freezer. Beat or process until a 'slush' forms. Return to the pan and freeze until firm. Remove from freezer 15–20 minutes before serving.

HINT:
• Sorbets may be served before the main course to refresh the palate, or with other creams or fruit as a dessert.

nutrition per serve: Energy 546 kJ (130 Cal); Fat 0.2 g; Saturated fat 0 g; Protein 0.6 g; Carbohydrate 30.8 g; Fibre 3.7 g; Cholesterol 0 mg; Sodium 7 mg

DAZZLE YOUR FRIENDS WITH THIS DELICIOUS SUNDAE. IT'S LOW GI AND KILOJOULES, AND BERRIES ARE PROVIDES GOOD AMOUNTS OF FIBRE AND ANTIOXIDANTS.

nutrition per serve: Energy 396 kJ (95 Cal)
Fat 1.7 g
Saturated fat 1 g
Protein 2.6 g
Carbohydrate 14.9 g
Fibre 3.9 g
Cholesterol 8 mg
Sodium 17 mg

MIXED BERRY SUNDAE WITH RASPBERRY CREAM

45 g (1¾ oz) sucralose
juice of 1 lemon
1 kg (2 lb 4 oz) mixed summer berries,
  including blueberries, loganberries,
  raspberries and strawberries
extra fresh berries, to serve

RASPBERRY CREAM
250 g (9 oz/2 cups) fresh raspberries
50 g (1¾ oz/½ cup) icing (confectioners')
  sugar

125 ml (4 fl oz/½ cup) extra-light thickened
  (whipping) cream

PREP TIME: 15 MINUTES + 7 HOURS
  FREEZING
COOKING TIME: NIL
SERVES 10

Put 500 ml (17 fl oz/2 cups) water in a saucepan and add the sucralose. Heat gently over low heat until the sucralose has dissolved. Bring to the boil, then reduce the heat and simmer for 5 minutes. Set aside to cool, then stir in the lemon juice.

Put the sweet syrup and mixed berries in a large processor fitted with the metal blade and blend for 20 seconds, or until smooth. Press the purée through a sieve in batches and pour into a wide, deep plastic container.

Freeze the mixture for 1–2 hours, or until ice crystals have formed around the edges. Using an immersion blender or blender, blend to break up the ice crystals. Return to the freezer and repeat this process for 4–5 hours until the berry mixture resembles soft snow. Remove from freezer 15–20 minutes before serving.

To make the raspberry cream, blend the raspberries and icing sugar in a small processor for 10 seconds, or until smooth. Press through a fine sieve. Lightly whip the cream until it just holds its shape. Fold the cream into the raspberry purée.

Serve the frozen sundae mixture in chilled glasses with a spoonful of raspberry cream and some fresh berries.

STEWED PEAR, APPLE AND RHUBARB WITH CUSTARD

A HEALTHY, LOW FAT TREAT FOR THE WHOLE FAMILY, THIS DESSERT IS LOADED WITH POTASSIUM, MANGANESE AND CALCIUM.

2 tbsp blackcurrant syrup
2 large pears, peeled, cored and quartered
1 apple, peeled, cored and quartered
500 g (1 lb 2 oz) rhubarb, trimmed, cut into
   3 cm (1¼ in) pieces
500 ml (17 fl oz/2 cups) skim milk

55 g (2 oz/¼ cup) caster (superfine) sugar
1½ tbsp custard powder

PREP TIME: 20 MINUTES
COOKING TIME: 20 MINUTES
SERVES 4

Put the syrup, pears, apple and 60 ml (2 fl oz/¼ cup) water in a large saucepan and stir to coat the fruits. Cook, covered, over low heat for 4 minutes, then add the rhubarb. Toss well to combine, then cover and cook for a further 6–7 minutes, or until the fruit is just tender. Remove from the heat, cover and leave to stand.

Put the milk and sugar in a saucepan. Bring to the boil, then reduce the heat and simmer for 3 minutes. Mix the custard powder with 1 tablespoon water to a smooth paste. Return the milk to the boil, stir in the custard powder mixture and whisk constantly until the mixture boils and thickens, and can coat the back of a wooden spoon.

Put the fruit in serving dishes and drizzle with any liquid from the bottom of the pan. Serve with the warm custard.

nutrition per serve: Energy 965 kJ (231 Cal); Fat 0.4 g; Saturated fat 0.2 g; Protein 5.8 g; Carbohydrate 50.5 g; Fibre 4 g; Cholesterol 4 mg; Sodium 65 mg

PEACH YOGHURT MOUSSE

THIS LIGHT DESSERT IS GREAT IN SUMMER WHEN PEACHES ARE IN SEASON. IT'S HIGH IN POTASSIUM AND PROVIDES SOME FIBRE AND CALCIUM.

125 g (4½ oz/1 cup) dried peaches
250 ml (9 fl oz/1 cup) peach nectar
2 tsp powdered gelatine
200 g (7 oz/¾ cup) reduced-fat plain yoghurt
2–3 tsp honey, to taste
3 egg whites

2 tbsp toasted flaked almonds, to serve

PREP TIME: 15 MINUTES + 1 HOUR REFRIGERATION
COOKING TIME: 10 MINUTES
SERVES 4

Put the peaches and peach nectar in a small saucepan. Cook over low heat, stirring often, for 10 minutes, or until the peaches are soft and pulpy. Set aside to cool for 10 minutes.

Put 2 tablespoons of hot water in a small bowl and sprinkle the gelatine over the top. Whisk with a fork for 1 minute, or until the gelatine has dissolved.

Put the peach mixture, gelatine mixture and yoghurt in a small processor or blender fitted with the metal blade. Process for 20–30 seconds, or until smooth. Add the honey, to taste, and blend to combine.

Whisk the egg whites until firm peaks form. Pour the peach mixture into the egg whites and gently fold through using a metal spoon.

Spoon the mousse into 4 x 250 ml (9 fl oz/1 cup) parfait glasses and smooth the surface. Cover and refrigerate for at least 1 hour, or until firm. Serve sprinkled with the almonds.

nutrition per serve: Energy 858 kJ (205 Cal); Fat 4.6 g; Saturated fat 0.8 g; Protein 9.7 g; Carbohydrate 29.2 g; Fibre 3.3 g; Cholesterol 5 mg; Sodium 84 mg

STICKY FIG AND HAZELNUT PUDDINGS

45 g (1½ oz/⅓ cup) hazelnuts
150 ml (5 fl oz) fresh orange juice
100 g (3½ oz/½ cup) chopped dried figs,
  plus 6 dried figs, extra, cut horizontally
¼ tsp ground ginger
¼ tsp ground cinnamon
3 tsp finely grated orange zest
½ tsp bicarbonate of soda (baking soda)
60 g (2¾ oz) canola margarine, softened
115 g (4 oz/½ cup) soft brown sugar

1 egg
90 g (3¼ oz/¾ cup) self-raising flour
2 tbsp maple syrup
boiling water, for steaming
low-fat vanilla custard or cream, to serve

PREP TIME: 25 MINUTES + 10 MINUTES
  COOLING TIME
COOKING TIME: 45 MINUTES
MAKES 6

Preheat the oven to 200°C (400°F/Gas 6). Spread the hazelnuts out on a tray and place in the oven for 6–7 minutes, until lightly toasted. Tip the nuts onto a clean tea towel (dish towel) and gently rub to remove the skins. Put the nuts in a food processor and pulse until finely ground. Grease six 250 ml (9 fl oz/1 cup) ramekins or ovenproof teacups and place a square of baking paper in the base of each.

Pour the orange juice into a saucepan and bring to the boil over medium heat. Add the chopped figs, ginger, cinnamon and 1 teaspoon of the orange zest and cook for 1 minute. Remove from the heat and add the bicarbonate of soda (allowing the mixture to froth), then set aside to cool for 10 minutes.

Meanwhile, combine the margarine and sugar in a large bowl and beat with electric beaters until light and fluffy. Add the egg and beat until well combined. Fold in the hazelnuts, and add the flour in three batches, incorporating each batch well into the mixture before adding the next (the mixture will become stiff). Pour the orange sauce into the pudding mixture and stir well to combine.

Pour the maple syrup into the base of the ramekins and top with the remaining orange zest. Arrange two of the extra fig halves in the base of each ramekin. Spoon in the pudding mixture until each ramekin is three-quarters full, then cover securely with a square sheet of foil. Arrange the puddings in the base of a deep roasting tin. Fill the baking tin with enough boiling water to come halfway up the sides of the ramekins, and bake the puddings for 35 minutes, or until cooked. Set the ramekins aside for 5 minutes before inverting onto a plate and serving with custard or cream.

THIS RECIPE IS A LOWER FAT
VERSION OF STICKY DATE
PUDDING, BUT ENJOY IN
MODERATION—IT'S NOT LOW
IN KILOJOULES.

nutrition per serve: Energy 1945 kJ (465 Cal)
Fat 14.2 g
Saturated fat 2.4 g
Protein 9.5 g
Carbohydrate 74 g
Fibre 6.6 g
Cholesterol 38 mg
Sodium 406 mg

171

COUSCOUS AND APRICOT PUDDINGS

A GOOD CHOICE FOR PEOPLE WITH HIGH BLOOD PRESSURE AS WELL AS HIGH
CHOLESTEROL—THIS DESSERT IS HIGH IN POTASSIUM AND LOW IN CHOLESTEROL.

90 g (3¼ oz/½ cup) dried apricots,
   chopped
875 ml (30 fl oz/3½ cups) apricot nectar
1 tbsp grated lemon zest
1 vanilla bean, split, seeds scraped
1 cinnamon stick
¼ tsp ground cloves
1 tbsp lemon juice

185 g (6½ oz/1 cup) couscous
low-fat vanilla custard, to serve

PREP TIME: 20 MINUTES
COOKING TIME: 45 MINUTES
SERVES 6

Grease six 250 ml (9 fl oz/1 cup) pudding bowls or ovenproof teacups and put a round of
baking paper in the bottom of each. Combine the apricots, nectar, lemon zest, vanilla bean
and seeds, and cinnamon stick in a saucepan over medium heat and bring to the boil.

Reduce the heat and simmer for 5 minutes, then remove from the heat and leave for
5 minutes. Strain, reserving the apricots and discarding the vanilla bean and cinnamon
stick. Return the nectar to the saucepan and divide the apricots among the pudding bowls.

Add the cloves, lemon juice and couscous to the reserved apricot nectar. Bring to the boil,
then reduce the heat to low and simmer, covered, for 8–10 minutes, or until most of the
liquid has been absorbed. The mixture should still be quite wet.

Spoon the couscous into the pudding bowls, level the top and cover each with a round of
foil. Place the bowls in a steamer and cover with a lid. Sit the steamer over a saucepan or
wok of boiling water and steam for 30 minutes, checking the water level regularly.

To serve, turn the puddings out of the bowls and serve hot with custard.

nutrition per serve: Energy 1353 kJ (323 Cal); Fat 1.4 g; Saturated fat 0.8 g; Protein 9.4 g;
Carbohydrate 67 g; Fibre 3.2 g; Cholesterol 7 mg; Sodium 69 mg

PEAR AND GINGER FILO PARCELS

THESE REDUCED-FAT PARCELS ARE A GREAT DESSERT TO SERVE AT A DINNER PARTY. THE PEAR PROVIDES POTASSIUM AND SOLUBLE FIBRE.

30 g (1 oz/¼ cup) flame raisins or other small seedless raisins

1 tbsp cognac or pear eau-de-vie

2 tsp lemon juice

3 Bosc pears

50 g (1¾ oz) ginger nut biscuits (ginger snaps), roughly broken

40 g (1½ oz/¼ cup) soft brown sugar

½ tsp mixed (pumpkin pie) spice

2 tbsp cornflour (cornstarch)

1 egg yolk

8 sheets filo pastry

canola oil spray

icing (confectioners') sugar, to serve

softened low-fat vanilla ice cream, to serve

PREP TIME: 30 MINUTES

COOKING TIME: 25 MINUTES

SERVES 4

Preheat the oven to 190°C (375°F/Gas 5). Line a baking tray with baking paper.

Put the raisins and liqueur in a small bowl and set aside. Put the lemon juice in a bowl. Peel, quarter and core the pears. Add them to the bowl and toss to coat with the lemon juice.

Put the ginger nut biscuits in a mini processor or blender and add the sugar, mixed spice and cornflour. Blend for 15 seconds, or until the mixture forms fine crumbs. Roughly chop half the pears and add to the processor. Add the egg yolk and blend in 2-second bursts for 15–25 seconds, or until the pears are chopped medium–fine. The mixture will be quite thin.

Cut the remaining pears into 2 cm (¾ in) dice and return to their bowl. Add the raisin mixture and processed pear mixture and toss to combine.

Lay a sheet of filo on a work surface and spray with oil. Fold in half, one short side over the other and spray with oil. Top with another sheet of filo, fold that in half and spray with oil, giving four layers of pastry. Trim the pastry to an 18 cm (7 in) square. Spoon one-quarter of the pear filling onto the centre. Starting at one corner, fold the filo over the filling to make a fat, square envelope. Ensure that the filling is well contained, and spray dry surfaces of the pastry as you fold. Spray the parcel all over with oil and place on the prepared tray, fold side up. Make three more parcels using the remaining pastry and filling.

Bake for 20–25 minutes, or until the parcels are crisp and golden. Serve hot, dusted with icing sugar and with a little softened vanilla ice cream spooned on top.

nutrition per serve: Energy 1683 kJ (402 Cal); Fat 7.3 g; Saturated fat 2.4 g; Protein 6.9 g; Carbohydrate 75.8 g; Fibre 3.8 g; Cholesterol 51 mg; Sodium 291 mg

THIS TASTY DISH IS READY IN A FLASH. IT HAS LESS FAT THAN TRADITIONAL CRUMBLES, BUT STILL HAS ALL THE FLAVOUR.

nutrition per serve: Energy 1048 kJ (250 Cal)
Fat 4.8 g
Saturated fat 1.5 g
Protein 4.7 g
Carbohydrate 46.1 g
Fibre 3.9 g
Cholesterol 5 mg
Sodium 91 mg

NECTARINE CRUMBLE WITH MAPLE AND LIME SYRUP

3 tbsp maple syrup
1 tsp finely grated lime zest
4 ripe nectarines, cut in half, stones
   removed
30 g (1 oz/¼ cup) self-raising flour
30 g (1 oz) light canola margarine
2 tbsp soft brown sugar
low-fat vanilla ice cream, to serve

PREP TIME: 20 MINUTES + 15 MINUTES
  INFUSING TIME
COOKING TIME: 5 MINUTES
SERVES 4

Put the maple syrup and lime zest in a bowl. Stir well and leave to infuse for 15 minutes.

Heat the grill (broiler) to medium. Lightly brush the cut side of the nectarine halves with some of the syrup. Put the nectarine halves, cut side down, in a lightly oiled non-stick frying pan. Gently fry over low–medium heat for 1 minute on each side, or until slightly soft.

Put the flour in a small bowl and add the butter. Using your fingertips, rub the butter into the flour until the mixture resembles breadcrumbs, then stir through the sugar.

Sit the nectarines on the grill tray, cut side up. Lightly brush them with a little more syrup, then sprinkle the crumble mixture over the top and grill for 2 minutes, or until the crumble turns golden brown. Divide among four serving bowls and drizzle with the remaining syrup. Serve with a scoop of low-fat vanilla ice cream.

REDUCED-FAT CHOCOLATE CAKE WITH STRAWBERRIES

WHO CAN SAY NO TO A SLICE OF CHOCOLATE CAKE? THIS VERSION HAS LESS FAT THAN TRADITIONAL CHOCOLATE CAKES BUT SHOULD BE ENJOYED IN MODERATION.

3 eggs

185 g (6½ oz/1 cup) lightly packed soft brown sugar

40 g (1½ oz) reduced-fat canola oil margarine, melted

170 ml (5½ fl oz/⅔ cup) ready-made apple sauce

60 ml (2 fl oz/¼ cup) skim milk

85 g (3 oz/⅔ cup) unsweetened cocoa powder

185 g (6½ oz/1½ cups) self-raising flour

strawberries, to serve

CHOCOLATE ICING

125 g (4½ oz/1 cup) icing (confectioners') sugar, sifted

2 tbsp unsweetened cocoa powder

1–2 tbsp skim milk

PREP TIME: 20 MINUTES

COOKING TIME: 40 MINUTES

SERVES 12

Preheat the oven to 180°C (350°F/Gas 4). Brush a 20 cm (8 in) kugelhopf tin with melted butter, dust lightly with flour and shake out any excess.

Whisk the eggs and sugar in a bowl for 5 minutes, or until pale and thick. Combine the margarine, apple sauce and milk in a small bowl, stirring to mix well, then fold into the egg mixture. Sift the cocoa powder and flour together into a bowl, then fold into the egg mixture.

Pour the mixture into the tin and bake for 35–40 minutes, or until a skewer inserted into the centre of the cake comes out clean. Leave the cake to cool in the tin for 5 minutes, then turn out onto a wire rack to cool completely.

To make the chocolate icing, combine the icing sugar and cocoa powder in a bowl, then stir in enough milk to form a thick paste. Stand the bowl over a saucepan of simmering water, stirring until the icing is smooth, then remove from the heat. Spread the icing over the cake and and arrange a few unhulled strawberries over the top. Hull and chop remainder of strawberries and serve with the cake.

This chocolate cake is best eaten on the day it is made.

nutrition per serve: Energy 978 kJ (234 Cal); Fat 4 g; Saturated fat 1.3 g; Protein 6 g; Carbohydrate 43.3 g; Fibre 2.3 g; Cholesterol 47 mg; Sodium 157 mg

PRUNE AND PECAN LOAF

THIS FRUIT LOAF IS DELICIOUS AND GREAT TO SERVE WHEN FRIENDS DROP BY FOR AFTERNOON TEA. IT'S A GOOD SOURCE OF FIBRE AND PROVIDES SOME ANTIOXIDANTS.

canola oil spray
60 g (2¼ oz) light canola margarine
80 g (2¾ oz/⅓ cup) raw sugar
1 tsp natural vanilla extract
250 g (9 oz/1 cup) chopped pitted prunes
60 g (2¼ oz/½ cup) pecans, chopped
250 g (9 oz/1⅔ cups) stoneground
  self-raising flour

1 tsp freshly grated nutmeg
60 g (2¼ oz/½ cup) unprocessed barley
  bran or oat bran

PREP TIME: 15 MINUTES
COOKING TIME: 45 MINUTES
MAKES 10–12 SLICES

Preheat the oven to 170°C (325°F/Gas 3). Spray a 19.5 x 9.5 cm (7½ x 3¾ in) loaf tin with oil, then line the base with baking paper.

Put the margarine, sugar, vanilla, chopped prunes and pecans in a large bowl. Pour over 250 ml (9 fl oz/1 cup) boiling water and stir to just melt the margarine.

Sift the flour and nutmeg into the bowl, then add the barley bran and return any husks to the bowl. Stir until well incorporated. Spoon into the prepared tin and smooth the surface.

Bake for 45 minutes, or until cooked when tested with a metal skewer. Cover with foil if the top is browning too much. Leave in the tin 10 minutes, then turn out onto a wire rack to cool. Cut into slices to serve. Serve warm or cold. Delicious toasted.

HINTS:
• Will keep refrigerated for up to 1 week, and frozen for up to 1 month.
• If you can't find barley bran in your supermarket, look for it at a health food shop.

nutrition per slice (12): Energy 879 kJ (210 Cal); Fat 6.2 g; Saturated fat 0.7 g; Protein 3.6 g; Carbohydrate 33.3 g; Fibre 3.8 g; Cholesterol 0 mg; Sodium 150 mg

CINNAMON, APPLE AND WALNUT CAKE

canola oil spray
250 g (9 oz/1⅔ cups) stoneground self-
   raising flour
2 tsp ground cinnamon
½ tsp baking powder
55 g (2 oz/½ cup) ground almonds
55 g (2 oz/¼ cup) caster (superfine) sugar
2 apples, peeled, cored and diced
60 g (2¼ oz/½ cup) chopped walnuts
2 eggs

125 ml (4 fl oz/½ cup) buttermilk
140 g (5 oz/½ cup) unsweetened apple
   purée
2 tbsp canola oil

PREP TIME: 20 MINUTES
COOKING TIME: 50 MINUTES
SERVES 10–12

Preheat the oven to 180°C (350°F/Gas 4). Spray a 23 cm (9 in) round cake tin with oil, then line the base with baking paper.

Sift the flour, cinnamon and baking powder into a large bowl, then return any husks to the bowl. Stir in the ground almonds and sugar, then the diced apple and chopped walnuts.

Whisk together the eggs, buttermilk, apple purée and oil in a bowl. Add to the flour mixture, then stir until combined and smooth. Spoon into the prepared tin and smooth the surface.

Bake for 50 minutes, or until cooked when tested with a metal skewer. Leave in the tin for 15 minutes, then turn out onto a wire rack to cool. Cut into wedges to serve. Delicious served warm.

HINT:
• Will keep refrigerated for up to 1 week. Freeze for up to 1 month.

THIS SPICED APPLE CAKE IS
GREAT COMFORT FOOD, IT CAN
BE SERVED WARM OR COLD.
ENJOY IN MODERATION.

nutrition per serve: Energy 916 kJ (219 Cal)
Fat 10.4 g
Saturated fat 1 g
Protein 5.4 g
Carbohydrate 25.1 g
Fibre 2.5 g
Cholesterol 32 mg
Sodium 194 mg

FRUIT AND TEA LOAF

THIS IS A GREAT LOW CHOLESTEROL TEA LOAF—IT DOESN'T CONTAIN ANY OIL
OR BUTTER. IT'S GOOD TO SERVE ANY TIME OF DAY.

500 g (1 lb 2 oz/2¾ cups) mixed dried fruit
185 ml (6 fl oz/¾ cup) strong, hot black tea
125 g (4½ oz/⅔ cup) lightly packed soft
   brown sugar
1 egg, lightly beaten
125 g (4½ oz/1 cup) plain (all-purpose)
   flour
¾ tsp baking powder
1 tsp ground cinnamon

¼ tsp ground nutmeg
a large pinch of ground cloves

PREP TIME: 20 MINUTES + 3 HOURS SOAKING
COOKING TIME: 1 HOUR 35 MINUTES
SERVES 10–12

Combine the fruit and hot tea in a large bowl, cover with plastic wrap and leave for 3 hours
or overnight. Preheat the oven to 160°C (315°F/Gas 2–3). Grease a 25 x 11 cm (10 x 4¼ in)
loaf tin and line the base with baking paper. Dust the sides of the tin with a little flour,
shaking off any excess.

Stir the sugar and egg into the fruit mixture and combine well. Sift the flour, baking
powder and spices into a bowl, then add the fruit mixture. Using a large slotted spoon, stir
to combine well.

Spoon the mixture into the tin and bake for 1 hour 35 minutes, covering the top with foil
if it browns too quickly. The loaf is cooked when a skewer inserted into the centre of the
loaf comes out clean. Cool the loaf in the tin, then turn out and serve, sliced and buttered,
if desired.

The loaf will keep, wrapped in plastic wrap and stored in an airtight container in a cool
place, for up to 1 week, or up to 8 weeks in the freezer.

nutrition per serve (12): Energy 834 kJ (199 Cal); Fat 1 g; Saturated fat 0.3 g; Protein 2.6 g;
Carbohydrate 45 g; Fibre 2.9 g; Cholesterol 16 mg; Sodium 86 mg

ITALIAN DRIED FRUIT BUNS

FOR A SPECIAL TREAT, WHY NOT PUT THE KETTLE ON AND GRAB ONE OF THESE TASTY BUNS. THEY'RE LOWER IN FAT THAN SCONES AND OTHER BUNS.

90 g (3¼ oz/¾ cup) raisins

3 tsp instant dried yeast

80 g (2¾ oz/⅓ cup) caster (superfine) sugar

400 g (14 oz/3 cups) strong flour

35 g (1¼ oz/¼ cup) unprocessed wheat or oat bran

1 tsp almond essence

1 tbsp olive oil

finely grated zest from 1 orange

40 g (1½ oz/¼ cup) mixed peel

40 g (1½ oz/¼ cup) pine nuts

1 egg, lightly beaten

115 g (4 oz/½ cup) caster (superfine) sugar, extra

PREP TIME: 30 MINUTES + 20 MINUTES SOAKING + 2 HOURS 50 MINUTES RISING TIME

COOKING TIME: 15 MINUTES

MAKES 12

Cover the raisins with 250 ml (9 fl oz/1 cup) boiling water in a small bowl and set aside for 20 minutes. Drain, reserving the liquid. Put half the liquid into a bowl, add the yeast, a pinch of the sugar and 30 g (1 oz/¼ cup) of the flour. Stir to combine, then leave in a draught-free place for 10 minutes, or until the yeast is foamy.

Add the remaining flour, bran, sugar and pinch of salt into the bowl of an electric mixer with a dough hook attachment and make a well in the centre. Combine the remaining raisin water with the almond essence and oil, then pour it, along with the yeast mixture, into the well. Add the raisins, orange zest, mixed peel and pine nuts. With the mixer set to the lowest speed, mix until a dough forms. Increase the speed to medium and knead the dough for 5 minutes, or until it is smooth and elastic; add a little more flour if necessary. Alternatively, mix the dough by hand using a wooden spoon, then turn out onto a floured work surface and knead for 10 minutes, or until smooth and elastic.

Grease a large bowl with oil, then transfer the dough to the bowl, turning the dough to coat in the oil. Cover with plastic wrap and leave to rise in a draught-free place for 2 hours, or until the dough has doubled in size. Knock back the dough by punching it gently, then turn out onto a lightly floured work surface. Divide the dough into 12 equal portions and shape each piece into an oval. To glaze the rolls, coat them in egg, then roll them in the extra sugar to coat. Transfer the rolls to a greased baking tray and leave for 30–40 minutes, or until the rolls have risen a little (they won't quite double in size). Meanwhile, preheat the oven to 200°C (400°F/Gas 6). Bake the rolls for 15 minutes, or until golden, then transfer to a wire rack to cool.

nutrition per serve: Energy 1112 kJ (266 Cal); Fat 5 g; Saturated fat 0.6 g; Protein 5.7 g; Carbohydrate 47.9 g; Fibre 3.2 g; Cholesterol 16 mg; Sodium 172 mg

THIS DELICIOUS FRUITY BREAD
IS LOW IN FAT AND MAKES AN
EXCELLENT LIGHT MEAL OR
SNACK. ENJOY ON ITS OWN OR
WITH A LOW-FAT TOPPING.

nutrition per serve (12): Energy 752 kJ (180 Cal)
Fat 0.9 g
Saturated fat 0.2 g
Protein 4.2 g
Carbohydrate 37.4 g
Fibre 3.9 g
Cholesterol 1 mg
Sodium 106 mg

APRICOT AND FIG BRAN BREAD

canola oil spray
110 g (3¾ oz/1 cup) unprocessed oat bran
250 ml (9 fl oz/1 cup) skim or no-fat milk
80 g (2¾ oz/½ cup) dried apricots,
    quartered
110 g (3¾oz/½ cup dried figs, quartered
185 g (6¼ oz/1 cup) soft brown sugar

150 g (5½ oz/1 cup) self-raising flour
1 tsp ground cinnamon

PREP TIME: 15 MINUTES + 10 MINUTES
    SOAKING TIME
COOKING TIME: 45 MINUTES
MAKES 1 LOAF (10–12 SLICES)

Preheat the oven to 180°C (350°F/Gas 4). Spray a 10 x 18 cm (4 x 7 in) loaf tin with the oil and line the base with baking paper.

Put the bran in a large bowl. Stir in the milk, dried fruit and sugar. Set aside for 10 minutes to soften the bran.

Meanwhile, sift the flour and cinnamon into a bowl. Stir the combined flour and cinnamon into the bran mixture. Pour into the prepared tin and bake for 45 minutes, or until cooked when a skewer inserted into the centre of the loaf comes out clean. Cool in the tin for 10 minutes, then turn out. Cut into thick slices to serve.

HINT:
• Leftovers of this loaf are delicious when toasted. You can freeze the loaf for up to 1 month. Use any 2–3 varieties of dried fruit or fruit medley in this recipe.

FRUIT MUFFINS

LOWER IN FAT AND KILOJOULES THAN MOST COMMERCIAL VARIETIES,
THESE TANGY MUFFINS ARE A GREAT SOURCE OF FIBRE, POTASSIUM
AND PHOSPHORUS.

160 g (5¾ oz/1 cup) chopped mixed dried
    fruit (apricots, dates, peaches or fruit
    medley with peel)
225 g (8 oz/1½ cups) wholemeal self-
    raising flour
1 tsp baking powder
150 g (5½ oz/1 cup) unprocessed oat bran
60 g (2¼ oz/⅓ cup) brown sugar

300 ml (10½ fl oz) skim milk
1 egg
1 tbsp oil

PREP TIME: 15 MINUTES + 5 MINUTES
    SOAKING
COOKING TIME: 20 MINUTES
MAKES 12

Preheat the oven to moderate 180°C (350°F/Gas 4). Grease twelve ½ cup (125 ml) muffin holes. Soak the dried fruit with 60 ml (2 fl oz/¼ cup) boiling water for 5 minutes.

Sift the flour and baking powder into a large bowl, returning the husks to the bowl. Stir in the oat bran and sugar and make a well in the centre.

Combine the milk, egg and oil in a jug. Add the soaked fruit and milk mixture all at once to the dry ingredients. Fold in gently using a metal spoon, until just combined—do not overmix.

Divide the mixture evenly among the muffin holes. Bake for 20 minutes, or until the muffins are risen and golden, and a skewer inserted into the centre comes out clean. Cool for a few minutes in the tin, then turn out onto a wire rack. Serve warm or at room temperature.

nutrition per muffin: Energy 805 kJ (192 Cal); Fat 3.3 g; Saturated fat 0.5 g; Protein 6.3 g; Carbohydrate 32.2 g; Fibre 5.1 g; Cholesterol 16 mg; Sodium 204 mg

APPLE AND PEACH MUFFINS

THESE MUFFINS ARE QUICK AND EASY TO MAKE AS THE INGREDIENTS ARE
ONLY LIGHTLY MIXED INSTEAD OF BEATEN SMOOTH. YOU CAN QUICKLY WHIP
UP A BATCH FOR A SPECIAL BREAKFAST OR AN AFTERNOON TREAT.

canola oil spray
150 g (5½ oz/1 cup) plain stoneground
   self-raising flour
80 g (2¾ oz/½ cup) wholemeal
   stoneground self-raising flour
1½ tsp ground cinnamon
½ tsp baking powder
50 g (1¾ oz/½ cup) rolled barley or oats
60 g (2¼ oz/⅓ cup) soft brown sugar
150 g (5½ oz/1 cup) dried peaches,
   chopped

1 large green apple, peeled, cored
   and finely chopped
1 egg
250 ml (9 fl oz/1 cup) skim milk
60 g (2¼ oz) reduced-fat canola margarine,
   just melted

PREP TIME: 20 MINUTES

COOKING TIME: 25 MINUTES

MAKES 12

Preheat the oven to 170°C (325°F/Gas 3). Spray twelve 80 ml (2½ fl oz/⅓ cup) muffin
holes with oil.

Sift the flours, cinnamon and baking powder into a large bowl, then return any husks
to the bowl. Stir in the rolled barley, brown sugar, chopped peaches and chopped apple.
Make a well in the centre.

Whisk together the egg, milk and melted margarine and stir into the flour mixture until
just combined. Do not overmix. Spoon evenly into the muffin holes.

Bake for 20–25 minutes, or until firm to touch and golden brown. Leave in the tin for
5 minutes, then turn out onto a wire rack to cool. Delicious served warm or cold.

HINTS:
• Will keep refrigerated for up to 5 days or frozen for up to 1 month.
• To lower the kilojoules and GI slightly, you can use half sucralose and half sugar instead
  of sugar only, but the end result will not be quite so light and fluffy.

nutrition per muffin: Energy 704 kJ (168 Cal); Fat 3.4 g; Saturated fat 1.1 g; Protein 4.5 g;
Carbohydrate 29 g; Fibre 3.2 g; Cholesterol 16 mg; Sodium 188 mg

Contact information

AUSTRALIA

National Heart Foundation of Australia
Phone: 02 6232 3800
Heart line: 1300 36 27 87
Web: www.heartfoundation.com.au

Heart Research Institute
145–147 Missenden Road
Camperdown NSW 2050
Phone: 02 8208 8900
Web: www.hri.org.au

NEW ZEALAND

National Heart Foundation of New Zealand
9 Kalmia St
Ellerslie, Auckland 1130
Phone: 09 571 9191
Web: www.nhf.org.nz

CANADA

Heart and Stroke Foundation of Canada
222 Queen St, Suite 1402
Ottawa, ON K1P 5V9
Phone: 613 569 4361
Web: www.heartandstroke.ca

UNITED KINGDOM

The British Heart Foundation
14 Fitzhardinge St
London W1H D6H
Phone: 020 7935 0185
Web: www.bhf.org.uk

USA

American Heart Association
727 Greenville Avenue
Dallas, Texas 75231
Phone: 1800 242 8721
Web: www.americanheart.org

INDEX